Handbook f
Rhythmical Einre
According to
Wegman/Hauschka

Edited by Monica Layer in collaboration with
Monika Fingado, Hermann Glaser,
Edelgard Grosse-Brauckmann, and Rolf Heine

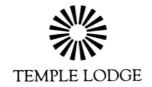

TEMPLE LODGE

To my teachers

Temple Lodge Publishing
Hillside House, The Square
Forest Row, RH18 5ES

www.templelodge.com

Published by Temple Lodge 2006

Originally published in German under the title *Praxishandbuch Rhythmische Einreibungen nach Wegman/ Hauschka* by Verlag Hans Huber, Bern, in 2003

This translation from the German contains some minor revisions to the original text at the authors' request

A catalogue record for this book is available from the British Library

ISBN-13: 978 1 902636 76 4
ISBN-10: 1 902636 76 7

Cover by Andrew Morgan Design
Typeset by DP Photosetting, Aylesbury, Bucks.
Printed and bound by Cromwell Press Limited, Trowbridge, Wilts.

Contents

Chapter 4

Note to the English Edition

Rhythmical Einreibung/en is a gentle rhythmical form of therapeutic massage used by nurses working out of anthroposophy. The word Einreibung is German for 'rubbing in', referring to the application of an oil or ointment to the body. Numerous attempts to find a suitable English word have been made, two such being 'embrocation' and 'oiling' which have been taken up in some countries. After a lot of discussion and consideration the British Anthroposophical Nurses Association has decided to continue to use the German word 'Einreibung/en' to represent this uniquely skilled and subtle form of massage carried out within professional guidelines.

Preface

Rhythmical Einreibungen according to Wegman/Hauschka, called Rhythmical Einreibungen in short, were developed at the beginning of the 20th century as a method for use in medicine and nursing extended through anthroposophy. They have become an important element in this approach and are used in hospitals, care homes and nursing homes, curative education and social therapy centres.

The method bears the names of the two physicians who pioneered this development, Dr Ita Wegman and Dr Margarethe Hauschka. Originally, physicians would mostly prescribe organ and whole-body Einreibungen as a medical treatment, sometimes doing the Einreibungen themselves. As time went on, Rhythmical Einreibungen became the responsibility of medical masseurs and masseuses and finally of nurses. For a long time, the method would be taught by medical masseurs and masseuses. It was only in the 1970s that nurses progressively took up the task of training. From then on, the use and teaching of Rhythmical Einreibungen as well as research have been largely in the hands of nursing professionals.

Gradually Rhythmical Einreibungen also came to be used for prophylaxis. This is an area where nurses are largely autonomous in establishing the indication and choosing suitable substances. For medical treatment Rhythmical Einreibungen with appropriate substances are specifically prescribed by physicians.

As with all external applications, it is important to work accurately and efficiently. We would not do full justice to the method, however, if we were to see it purely as an interesting nursing technique. It calls for clearly established goals and a rhythmical way of working and in addition for creativity and spontaneity on the nurse's part to give the Rhythmical Einreibungen skilfully, i.e. in accordance with the individual situation.

A Rhythmical Einreibung always calls for involvement of the carer's whole person. It does affect quality; for instance, how far a carer is able to make her own body (hands, body posture) so mobile that it will follow her intentions. It also matters considerably how far a carer is able to create an atmosphere of calm in and around herself and to make contact with the other person. The (simple) fact of warm or cold hands is another factor which has a major influence on the effectiveness of a Rhythmical Einreibung.

Other requirements for Rhythmical Einreibungen done with real skill are a good physical constitution, an ability to relate, expert knowledge, observance of quality criteria, which calls for careful technique. Rhythmical Einreibungen may thus also be seen as contributing to the inner personal and professional development of the carer. The competence needed personally and in social communication can be achieved and developed further by overcoming habits of thinking and physical and behavioural attitudes that may in part have become habit.

No claim is made that the book offers a representative overview of the Rhythmical Einreibungen 'landscape'. Different directions have developed since they were first used in the 1920s, with people using variations of the method. Each 'direction' is endeavouring to find the best possible way of using the rhythmical element in the procedure. The information and instructions given in this book should therefore be seen as a kind of 'snapshot'.

The aim in producing the book has been to give support in learning and teaching the method of Rhythmical Einreibungen. It is intended for everyone who

- wishes to use Rhythmical Einreibungen in their professional work and to review, extend or deepen their knowledge
- has attended introductory courses and wishes to read up on specific subject areas or find suggestions for going more deeply into the matter

- teaches Rhythmical Einreibungen and is looking for suggestions or further ideas.

As part of quality assurance, the International Further Training Council of Anthroposophical Care Professions has produced a valid and binding requirements profile for those who teach Rhythmical Einreibungen.

Concerning the contents of this book. Basic knowledge is required for independent, professional use of the Rhythmical Einreibungen according to Wegman/Hauschka. Chapter 1 briefly describes the aspects of the anthroposophical image of the human being that are most important in the context. Concepts which are important for the application and effectiveness of Rhythmical Einreibungen are introduced and explained. Some of the many aspects of the complex subject are briefly outlined.

In Chapter 2 clear distinction is made between rhythmical massage and Rhythmical Einreibungen. Details are given of how the rhythmical quality is created for the Einreibungen. General aspects concerning the use of different substances and the use of Rhythmical Einreibungen complete the chapter.

Chapter 3 begins with a description of the 'technique' of the part and organ Einreibungen which are most important in nursing. The points of view given in Chapter 2 are taken as read here, with no special reference made to them. One particular variant of Rhythmical Einreibungen is the Pentagram Einreibung. General aspects of a basic nature relating to this are included in the chapter.

The last Chapter offers specific exercises which can be used to develop the special skills required for the procedure. The exercises may also be used in training courses.

Acknowledgements

A heart-felt thank-you to everyone who has had a part in producing this book. Primarily these are the colleagues whose commitment during all the years of teaching and practising the Rhythmical Einreibungen has contributed to their application, understanding and further development. Apart from the practical work I am also thinking of the many intensive discussions at group meetings or in further and additional training courses. All those talks served to clarify and develop the theory and practice of Rhythmical Einreibungen. Without this valuable commitment it would not have been possible to publish at the present time.

A special thank-you to the many colleagues and friends not mentioned here by name who have made valuable suggestions, having studied the drafts in depth and with a critical eye. It is only thanks to all these people that it has been possible to put in writing everything those 'great ladies', Dr Ita Wegman and Dr Margarethe Hauschka, gave to the world with their Rhythmical Einreibungen, and so give a further impulse for the further development of these applications.

Personally I am especially indebted to E. Grosse-Brauckmann who has given me tremendous support, tirelessly and most thoroughly correcting and adding especially to Chapter 3.

Monika Layer
CH-Waengi
July 2002

Additional Acknowledgements
The translation of this book has been enabled by funds given by the British Anthroposophical Nurses Association (A.N.A.).

The A.N.A. would like to thank Edelgard Grosse-Brauckmann for her many inspiring courses given over the years, and Fiona Sim and Joan Smith for their hard work in bringing this publication to completion.

Chapter 1
Basic principles
Monika Layer

Rudolf Steiner established anthroposophy (wisdom of the human being) as a science of the spirit at the end of the 19th and beginning of the 20th centuries. He investigated the immaterial, non-physical in both human beings and the natural world, using scientific methods in a way that is comparable to the study of material things in natural science. In his fundamental epistemological works he described his concept of science, or his approach to scientific method. This does not differ from the method used in modern science, except that the field of investigation is extended to include the immaterial.

Steiner published many works and gave numerous lectures in which he described the realm of the immaterial and its laws in considerable detail. Different approaches to and instructions for inner development also show that every modern individual may gain personal insight into that realm by taking up these studies.

To progress from practice that is mere imitation to one based on real understanding, it is essential to study the roots of these external applications in the anthroposophical view of the human being. A brief description is therefore given in this chapter of the essential basic principles.

Some readers may find the anthroposophical view of the human being and the world rather different from anything they have known so far. Some general comments on how to work with them may therefore be indicated. For as long as one is not yet able to relate the subject matter to personal experience, getting to know about it is like reading a travelogue about a country which one would like to visit. You are greatly interested in that country but have not got your own ideas about it. As a reader you are nevertheless perfectly able to understand the report and take a critical view of the degree to which it reflects reality or probability. Reading about it may even make you want to add to what you have read and gain personal experience by going there. My advice would be to approach the results of Rudolf Steiner's investigations in this way. You may not have personal experience of the immaterial, but readers and health-care providers are asked to bring their unprejudiced thinking and unbiased powers of observation to this. Everyone can then form their own opinion, taking a critical view of the subject matter, and perhaps also feel encouraged to make their own investigations.

1   The human being in body, soul and spirit

In anthroposophy, the human being is seen as an integral whole made up of body, soul and spirit who is in interaction with the surrounding natural world that has arisen through evolution. The whole is differentiated in itself and has inner cohesion.

The living body serves soul and spirit as an instrument and an organ for coming to expression. The physical, material body is kept alive by a separate organization of powers, the 'ether body' or 'life body'. This also provides for growth and regeneration in the body. Section 2, on the four bodies, gives a detailed description of the relationship between physical body and ether body, this being of major importance for the understanding and practice of the Rhythmical Einreibungen.

The soul holds the living inner world of the human being. It encompasses all feelings, drives, instincts and passions, thoughts and will impulses. The soul mediates between individual and surrounding world. Its powers of thinking, feeling and will establish the relationship between inner and outside world in the gaining of insight, making of experiences, and giving direction to our actions.

Similar to the way in which it takes up impulses from the body and reacts to them (known from psychosomatic medicine), the soul also takes up impulses from the human spirit and reacts to them. It thus holds a middle position between spirit and body and acts as a mediator between these two planes.

The spiritual part of the human being has all bodily processes and all development at soul level to serve it during life. All functions are subservient to it, and it is the basis of human integrity. 'Spirit' in this human context means the 'I', the 'individual', the unique core which gives every human being a personal individual nature. This individual spirit is eternal, living in a physical body during life on earth, leaving it on death, and returning to earth again after a period in the world of the spirit.

During life on earth the individual seeks to develop the intentions brought from the world of the spirit, and so let his individual nature come to realization. J. W. Goethe took up this thought in a poem entitled *Urworte, orphisch* (Ancient Words, Orphic).

As the Sun stood, open to the hail of planets,
upon that day which gave you to the world
the way was set which you then followed,
true to the law of that beginning.
Thus you must be, unable to escape;
thus did Sibyls speak and prophets once,
and neither time nor might will break
the form once cast as it now lives and grows.

Wie an dem Tag, der dich der Welt verliehn
Die Sonne stand zum Grusse der Planeten
Bist alsobald und fort und fort gediehn
Nach dem Gesetz, wonach du angetreten.
So musst du sein, dir kannst du nicht entfliehn
so sprachen schon Sibyllen und Propheten
und keine Zeit und keine Macht zerstückelt
geprägte Form, die lebend sich entwickelt.

The I, incarnating on earth and letting body and soul serve it, reveals itself according to its own inherent laws. These become visible in a human biography. In the view taken of the human being in anthroposophy, the developmental steps which are part of the biography depend not only on hereditary disposition and external influences. Body, soul and spirit influence one another and this permits perfectly appropriate developmental steps to occur at the different stages of life (see under The four bodies, 2).

Developmental steps may follow 'normal' biographical development, but they may also be due to strokes of destiny, to sickness, accidents, social conflict or profound human encounters. In this sense these triggering factors help us to question established views, habits and values, which then opens up possibilities for starting again and making changes. Developmental steps, be they part of 'normal' biographical evolution or crisis-determined, are necessary if the individual (Goethe's 'law of that beginning') is to bring himself progressively to realization in accordance with the intentions of the I ('Thus you must be, unable to escape'). The I looks for and creates the bodily, psychological and social conditions that will help it to achieve this.

These conditions include

1   the parents, who provide the bodily preconditions by means of heredity
2   the social environment (family, teachers, friends, etc.), offering opportunities for important human encounters
3   the culture (country, language and religion) into which we are born, and
4   the age in which we live.

Within the framework thus created, it is then open to every individual to make his own decisions, which may well diverge from the routes embarked on before birth. People thus are not unfree, forced to adhere to 'guidelines' set before birth and to shape life accordingly. Human beings are indeed made for freedom, and it is for themselves to decide on the extent to which they take this up.

After death, the I lives on in the world of the spirit, going through an extended period of development. The past life on earth is looked at and evaluated, and this provides the basis for 'conceiving' a new life. The individual spirit then begins to prepare for a further cycle of life on earth and another incarnation.

Rudolf Steiner gave exact descriptions of this development after death and before birth. He described how destiny is created and the role which a human life on earth plays in this process. He showed how the consequences of everything done in one life are brought home again in the next. The events of a life, a person's attitude to tasks that have to be faced and to other people all play a crucial role in human development. In anthroposophy, the thought of reincarnation is therefore absolutely central to understanding the human being and human life.

1.1   The carer's attitude

The above outline of the image of the human being forms a basis for finding new answers to important questions in life, such as how to deal with sickness, strokes of destiny and disabilities, and with issues such abortion, genetic engineering and euthanasia. The thought of reincarnation can open up a new dimension for nurses, physicians, therapists and those who are directly affected, and may make it possible to find new ways of dealing with sickness, disability and death.

Nurses are at the side of their patients on the physical and also the psychological and spiritual planes. On the basis of the anthroposophical image of the human being, the aim in caring for those in need of care will be to do everything in one's power, working with the whole therapeutic team, to support the individual and maintain quality of life, so that he may proceed with dignity.

Caring for someone who is sick, disabled, old or dying, we go part of their way with them. In everything we do, every gesture, every conversation, everything, therefore, that is part of nursing care, we are at the service of that person. This basic attitude makes us into a vessel through which the individual patient receives a living impulse from the world of the spirit.

Conscious awareness in working with the principle of life, respect for the individual spirit and for the freedom of the other person, and knowledge of the relationship between man and nature are therefore central aspects in this approach to nursing. It adds a spiritual dimension to the familiar holistic approaches.

This wholeness in the approach also applies to quite practical aspects, for it has visible consequences in everyday nursing care. These aspects range from body care, external applications and conversation all the way to human relationships with patients and the nature of our collaboration in an organization. This 'practical wholeness of approach' provides us with instruments and methods which we can bring to our daily work.

One of these instruments or methods is the Rhythmical Einreibungen. In the chapters that follow, it will be shown how these aspects determine the way we act.

Sources

Heine R, Bay F (ed.). *Anthroposophische Pflegepraxis*. 2. Aufl. Stuttgart: Hippokrates 2001.

Steiner R. *Theosophy. An Introduction to the Spiritual Processes in Human Life and in the Cosmos*. Tr. C. E. Creeger. Hudson: Anthroposophic Press 1994.

Steiner R. *Manifestations of Karma*. Tr., 4th rev. edn London: Rudolf Steiner Press 1995.

Further reading

Lievegoed B. *Man on the Threshold*. Tr. Stroud: Hawthorn Press.

Lievegoed B. *Lebenskrisen Lebenschancen. Die Entwicklung des Menschen zwischen Kindheit und Alter*. 5. Aufl. Munich: Koesel 1986.

Steiner R. *The Philosophy of Freedom. A Philosophy of Spiritual Activity* (GA 4). Tr. R. Stebbing. London: Rudolf Steiner Press 1988. Also as *Intuitive Thinking as a Spiritual Path*. Tr. M. Lipson. Hudson: Anthroposophic Press 1995.

Steiner R. *An Outline of Esoteric Science* (GA 13). Tr. C. E. Creeger. Hudson: Anthroposophic Press 1997. Alternative translation: *Occult Science – An Outline*. Tr. G. & M. Adams. London: Rudolf Steiner Press 1962–3.

Steiner R. *The Forming of Destiny and Life after Death* (GA157a). Tr. H. Collison. London: Anthroposophical Publishing Co. 1927.

Steiner R. *Von Seelenraetseln* (GA 21). 5. Aufl. Dornach: Rudolf Steiner-Nachlassverwaltung 1983. Extracts in *The Case for Anthroposophy*. Tr. O. Barfield. London: Rudolf Steiner Press 1970.

Treichler R. *Soulways: The developing soul – Life phases, thresholds and biography*. Tr. A. R. Meuss. Stroud: Hawthorn Press.

2   The four bodies

2.1   General

In his anthroposophy, Rudolf Steiner described the human being as an integral whole made up of material and immaterial elements of body, life, soul and spirit. The anthroposophical differs from the conventional scientific view by accepting that the human *body* has not only material but also non-material parts. These are the bridge which allows soul and I/individual spirit to be present in an earthly body and live on earth.

If human beings were a conglomerate of nothing but material parts, they would be a lifeless machine. Yet like plants, human beings show the typical characteristics of life – growth, self healing and reproduction. These vanish when death ensues, and the lifeless mineral body then follows the laws of the material of which it is made. It dissolves. During life, dissolution is continually prevented by the activity of specific vital powers that organize different forms of matter in time and space in ways that are typical of life forms. These specific vital powers are referred to as the *ether body* or *life body*.

Unlike plants, humans and animals have not only life but also conscious awareness. A life form endowed with soul develops an inner life of its own, responding to impressions from the outside world with sentience, pain, pleasure, inclination, disinclination, desire, passions, etc. Such feelings and sensations can be given visible expression in actions and behaviour. The specific organization of powers which creates the basis for conscious awareness and soul life is referred to as the *astral body*.

Unlike animals, human beings are able to develop not only conscious awareness but also self awareness. They are not helplessly at the beck and call of anything they live through and encounter in their feelings but can bring their experiences to (self) awareness, be rational about them, and so give them direction and form. This is possible through the activity of

their self-aware spirit, the I. The organization of powers at its disposal is called the *I-organization*; this allows the I to be effective in the living body.

These four 'bodies' of the human being, briefly outlined above, form a hierarchy among themselves. The I-organization is the 'owner of the building', the highest authority in charge of all processes. The other three bodies are there to serve it.

As a help towards better understanding, the characteristic qualities of the four bodies are described below in terms of the 'elements', these being the four elements of ancient Greek philosophy. To the Greeks, the elements were divine in origin, mediating between the spiritual and earthly worlds. Natural philosophers such as Heraclitus or Thales of Miletus called them the 'original substance' out of which the earth is created. All natural phenomena could be shown to derive from them. The Greeks thus did not look at the elements in the way we do in physics or chemistry today. For them, they were connected with qualities of soul and spirit.

Today the best way of gaining insight into the Greek way of seeing these things is to let the qualities of the elements come alive in us and also apply them at the level of soul and spirit. Four fundamental qualities arise on unbiased observation, and we find them above all in the natural world (Table 1.1).

Below, the characteristic qualities of the elements are considered as a first step in describing one of the bodies. Try and let these qualities come alive before the inner eye by inwardly entering into natural processes you have observed, moods or other things in life that come close to the qualities of the elements or correspond to them fully. Visualize these processes in as much detail as possible. At the same time try to be aware of feelings arising in you in connection with these images, for they will give you an impression of the inner qualities of the elements. Letting them thus come inwardly alive in you creates a bridge to the qualities of the four bodies.

Table 1.1	The four bodies and the natural worlds			
Body	Basis for	Natural world	Element	Quality
I-organization	self awareness	human being	fire	heat that transforms
astral body	consciousness	animal	air	dynamics to give form
ether body	life	vegetable	water	flowing movement
physical body	matter	mineral	earth	resting solid state

2.2   Earth

The qualities of the physical body show themselves clearly if we compare it to the element 'earth', or the solid state of aggregation. A crystal occupies a space with definite boundaries, is rigid, immobile, and cannot change its established form of its own accord. It is primarily subject to the laws of mechanics. A crystal can only grow when material is added from outside; it cannot grow actively. The form is laid down and can only change if the consistency or concentration of the solution in which the crystal is growing changes. Crystals show the qualities of the inorganic, lifeless.

The element earth conveys security and support thanks to its qualities; it gives firmness.

Earth — how fast it stands!
Letting itself be tormented!
How people scratch and harrow it!
How they scarify and hoe it!
That is the way to go.
Making furrows and lines
All along its back,
Farm hands sweat over it;
And where no flowers bloom
It gets the blame.
From *Pandora*, by J. W. Goethe

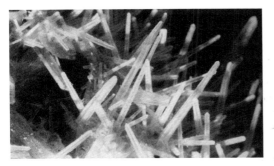

Fig. 1.1   Rock crystal (from Kniebe G. *Die vier Elemente*. Stuttgart: Freies Geistesleben 1993).

Erde sie steht so fest!
Wie sie sich quälen lässt!
Wie man sie scharrt und plackt!
Wie man sie ritzt und hackt!
Da soll's heraus.
Furchen und Striemen ziehn
Ihr auf den Rücken hin
Knechte mit Schweissbemühn;
Und wo nicht Blumen blühn,
Schilt man sie aus.
From *Pandora*, by J. W. Goethe

2.3.   The physical body

The physical body includes all the bodily structures we know from our study of anatomy. It is made up of substances or elements which also make up the inorganic world of nature — minerals, metals, oxygen, carbon, hydrogen, nitrogen, etc. We can touch and see the human physical body. It is a form in space and we can carry, perceive or move it. The laws active in it are above all those of physics.

The physical body includes everything that belongs to the solid, substantial basis of the human being. It is closely related to the mineral world, or the element earth, and therefore also to the inorganic. It is the instrument for all higher functions — those of life, soul and human spirit. Solidity prevails in it, and also a tendency to endure. According to Fintelmann, 'we must think of all solid tissue or organs as belonging (to the physical body), above all the tissues of nerves, sense organs and bones, but also all connective and supportive tissues' [V. Fintelmann 1987].

2.3.1   The physical body in the course of life

At the beginning of life, the structures belonging to the infant's physical body are still soft and in some parts undifferentiated. It is above all the skeleton which only grows solid in the early years, as it develops its function to hold and support. The tendency to harden increases especially in old age, when the tissues concerned lose elasticity and thus partly also their ability to function.

2.4   Water

Water has from time immemorial always been considered the vehicle for life. It was venerated and used in religious rites in all the early civilizations. In antiquity, the idea was that in water the sacred powers of heaven continue on earth. Water was considered to be the life-giving element, with the qualities of flowing movement inherent in it.

The physical and chemical properties of water are evident in many different phenomena in the natural world. It is capable of change and maintains a rhythmical balance between crystallization and dissolution. It can dissolve the salt of earth and take in the powers of light and heat. Interplay with earth and wind and the cosmic powers of sun and moon makes rhythms appear. It is to water that we owe the play of waves, for instance, the meanders of a river, ebb and flood, the constant alternation of evaporation and precipitation.

The element water is highly mobile and capable of change in its interplay with the other elements. It quickens and enlivens and is the precondition for all organic life.

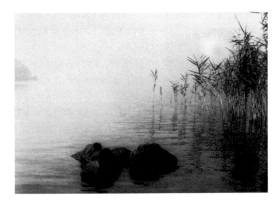

Fig. 1.2   Water.

Water, let it but flow!
Flowing by nature
From rocks down through fields,
It draws to its course
Both people and cattle.
Fishes in shoals so dense,
Birds in their flocks go hence –
Theirs is the flood.
Inconstant,
Stormy, alive,
A reasoning mind
May sometimes tame it,
Which we think is good.

        From *Pandora*, by J. W. Goethe

Wasser es fließe nur!
Bließet es von Natur
Felsenab durch die Flur,
Zieht es auf seine Spur
Menschen und Vieh.
Fische sie wimmeln da,
Vögel sie himmeln da,
Ihr' is die Flut.
Diue unbeständige
Stürmisch lebendige,
Dass der Verständige
Manchmal sie bändige,
Finden wir gut.

        From *Pandora*, by J. W. Goethe

2.5   The ether body

As the name indicates, the ether or life body is responsible for the processes belonging to the sphere of life. It is present throughout the physical body, pulsing through it, builds up its substances, keeps it in life, provides for growth, regeneration and reproduction. These are the powers that give human beings health or maintain them in health.

The ether body is a separate and specific system of powers that is not perceptible to the senses. Its effects can, however, be observed. The watery element enables the ether body to take effect in the organism, for all the properties of the watery element together make it the ideal vehicle for vital processes.

The etheric forces or powers are constructive by nature, configuring and shaping the body. They are considered to be the 'architect' and 'sculptor' of the living body. All life forms, including plants and animals, have an ether body.

In human beings, the etheric forces have the function of creating the body in conjunction with the other three bodies and they also have other tasks. They sustain memory, for instance. Everything we meet and learn in life leaves its imprint in the ether body. It is also the vehicle for our habits. Everyone who has ever tried it knows how difficult it is to change a habit once it has become established. The difficulty arises because habits are inscribed in the ether body, as it were, and therefore have to be 're-written' in active processes of the conscious mind. Habits can only be successfully changed once this has been done.

The powers of the ether body

1 enliven the physical body
2 provide for its nutrition, growth and regeneration
3 sustain habits and memory, and
4 are predominantly active in the metabolic sphere.

2.5.1 Gravity and levity

Like all mineral bodies, the physical body is subject to gravity. In water, levity cancels this to some extent. Levity as a force that acts against gravity is thus one of the qualities of water. Levity is active in the whole human water organism, overcoming a good part of gravity. This can be seen particularly well in the brain, which is wholly embedded in cerebrospinal fluid and thus also completely taken into levity.

If the relationship between gravity and levity is upset in the human body, feelings of discomfort will tend to arise that may develop into actual sickness. If you wake up after a good night's sleep – the ether body works with particular intensity during the night, taking care of regeneration – you feel fresh and light. After a strenuous day you feel tired at night, and adults will quite often also complain of swollen legs. This swelling and tiredness are due to the fact that the ether body

has partly withdrawn from the body so that physical forces predominate. The result is that our body fluids become partly subject to gravity.

In a healthy person this will have gone after a good night's rest. In ill health, night-time regeneration may not happen or be inadequate. Sick people will often complain of heaviness in the limbs in the mornings, feeling that they have not had enough sleep, or their legs may still be swollen. These are indications that the ether body has been unable to achieve regeneration during the night.

2.5.2 The ether body in the course of life

The etheric forces work in different ways in the human organism in the course of time. In the first seven years of life the ether body is particularly active in the growth and development of the child's body. Once the second teeth develop, the intensity lessens. The vital energies no longer needed for work on the body then serve to develop intellectual powers. The child will be ready for school and begins to develop an inner thought world of his or her own by learning to read, write and do sums.

Interest awakens in things outside one's own world, and children are increasingly more open to other spheres of life. After further developmental steps in the soul sphere, which will be considered later, the young person reaches adult age.

The middle period of adult life is a period of healthy equilibrium, with body-bound and body-free ether forces in balance. After the childhood diseases with their strong evolution, the adult lives through a phase of relative health until the early forties are reached.

With advancing age, from about the 40th year onwards, the vital energies withdraw more and more from the physical body. The health problems of old age then begin to arise. This separation of ether forces from the physical body enables human beings to take a further great step in development. Interests and personal concerns intensify, and people are able to consider their very own goals in life and essential, existential needs. In the ideal case, this reorientation will bring increasing wisdom and goodness as a person gets older.

The ageing/old person will, however, have to come to terms more and more with the ether forces that are becoming free. Apart from bodily symptoms this may also mean increasing inability to remember everyday things or even complete disorientation.

2.6   Air

The properties of the airy element are elasticity and dynamism. Something which is airy is able to take up other gases without needing additional space. Gases are thus able to reduce the space they occupy enormously under growing pressure. Excessive pressure may then 'give vent' to an explosion. Mobility and thorough mixing, condensing and dilution are characteristic qualities. They may be taken for an image of processes in which the human soul is living all the time. Wind with its dynamic properties became the image of inner change and new beginning for many poets, waking up dreamers and asking them to give new order and form to their lives.

The airy element is dynamic and creates tension. (Plate, Figure 1)

Wind, oh my friend!
For so long,
grey mountains hemmed me in.
Now I am free to welcome you again,
and you too are free;
child of heaven, give me again
sacred gift,
rousing sleepers from their rest
as you do.
Wind, o my friend!
Best companion of all!

                    Christian Morgenstern

Wind, du mein Freund!
Lang hielten Berge mich grämlich umzäunt.
Nun wieder grüss ich dich,
frei, dich, den Freienl;
nun gib mir, Himmelsspross,
wieder die Weihen,
Wecker zu sein wie du
Aller Verschlafenen Ruh!

Wind, du mein Freund!
Du mein liebster Genoss!

                    Christian Morgenstern

2.7   The astral body

It is harder to develop an understanding for the organization of astral powers than it is to grasp the ether body. Compared to the latter, which is active in the whole of the watery, living organization, the astral body acts in different ways in different organs and organ systems. This differentiated way of working calls for an equally differentiated approach to its study. Only brief reference can be made here to what is in fact a very complex matter.

In principle, the astral body opposes the continuously growing and developing powers of the ether body with powers that configure and create form by breaking down old forms.

Astral body activity

1   allows conscious awareness to develop
2   leads to locomotion, in which both animals and humans differ from the plant world
3   provides the basis for the life of the soul.

The astral body needs the airy element for its activities in the human organism. The air organism concentrates mainly on the cavities which make up the respiratory system but also includes the frontal and paranasal sinuses and the anterior part of the auditory system.

2.7.1   The astral body in the course of life

The work of the astral body in configuring the organs largely comes to an end with sexual maturity. Just as the organ-developing work of the etheric forces is completed after about seven years, so that they are then available for the development of thought life, so are the astral powers released from their organ-configuring task after about 14 years and then available for the development of a differentiated inner life.

Astral body activity breaks down or transforms etheric and physical forces. In early adulthood the process gets to be less dominant, but from the 40th year onwards the involutional process becomes increasingly evident in the signs of ageing. As mentioned above, the etheric forces begin to separate from the physical body at about this time, which happens in accordance with developmental laws. It will then depend on maturity and on the experiences a person has lived through to what extent he will be able to take hold of the powers which are thus released with his I and make them serve the impulses he has for life. The potential for this would at this age be available on the basis of purely 'physiological' processes.

2.8   Fire

Unlike the other elements, heat has played a major role in the development of cultural life. Human beings were only able to create the conditions for working with the other realms of nature once they had learned the effective use of fire.

Heat is present in all forms of matter, changing the state of substances. It brings movement into them and is thus the cause of their transformation. It makes air flow, water evaporate and metals melt. Physically, heat causes the other elements, especially the solid and fluid, to change to other states of aggregation. (Plate, Figure 2)

The image of heat, or warmth, will only be complete with reference to the human being if we also consider its soul dimension. Warmth means comfort and ease. Its absence (cold–frost) and an excess of it (heat–fire) lead to destruction and annihilation of life, causing unease and aloofness in the inner life. If we warm to an idea, developing enthusiasm for it, the life of thought influences the will and we do something. Anything which leaves us 'cold', being of no interest, will have no further consequences for us. To develop an interest and indeed to marvel at things are warmth processes transformed into soul qualities.

Ecce homo
Yes, I know whence I come!
Like an ever hungry flame
I burn, consuming self.
Alight comes all I touch,
charred is all I leave behind:
Flame I am for sure!
Friedrich Nietzsche

Ecce Homo
Ja, ich weiß, woher ich stamme!
Ungesättigt gleich der Flamme
Glühe und verzehr ich mich.
Licht wird alles, was ich fasse,
Kohle alles, was ich lasse:
Flamme bin ich sicherlich!
Friedrich Nietzsche

2.9   The I-organization

The I-organization is the basis and hence precondition for the fact that an individual is actually able to be in a (material) body. All other processes are subordinate to it and serve a goal which is to enable the incarnating individual to develop in soul and spirit. The I-organization thus is the bodily aspect of the I, being very closely connected with it.

Warmth is differentiated in the human being, which is also why we speak of a warmth organism. The differentiation can be perceived from the differences in temperature in different organ systems and diurnal variations in temperature. The I-organization establishes differentiated temperature regulation so that the body temperature may be maintained as required in different organs and organ systems. The regulation serves mainly the I, which depends on a constant core temperature of 36.5–37.5 °C for its governing functions. Even minor increases or decreases result in the clouding of consciousness.

The importance of warmth for the (bodily) I-organization and hence the presence of the (spiritual) I in the human organism cannot be rated too highly. It must be a central issue for health carers to take appropriate measures to support the warmth organism which generally tends to be affected during periods of sickness.

2.9.1 The warmth organism in the course of life

Warmth regulation is still imperfect in the newborn. They will thus get hot or chilled more easily due to external influences than adults do. Care must therefore be given to warmth states when looking after infants and young children.

The warmth organism grows more differentiated in childhood and youth, it gets stabilized and the violent febrile diseases of that age will gradually cease. In adults, warmth regulation is generally well balanced.

Old people gradually lose the ability to generate sufficient warmth and 'order' it in the body. The phenomenon may be considered to indicate that the I-organization, too, gradually separates from the body, and particularly from the metabolic sphere. This is a vast field in caring for the elderly. It needs to be developed further and perfected. Disease processes also have more of a 'cold' character in old age.

2.10 The four bodies and Rhythmical Einreibungen

The human being's four bodies have a hierarchic relationship, with the 'higher' always superior to the 'lower' one below it. Sickness arises when the relationship has grown inharmonious. Disorders develop especially in the connection and relationship between ether body and astral body.

With the Rhythmical Einreibungen we are, of course, working on the (material) human body, but we are more or less directly also working on etheric processes, astral processes, and processes of the I-organization.

The aim of the Rhythmical Einreibungen is to (re)establish a harmonious relationship between the bodies. Above all we seek to support the health-giving activities of the ether body, so that the I-organization may take effect. We therefore use all the qualities characteristic of the different bodies – solid, fluid, dynamic and warming. These qualities govern the whole approach, both for the actual treatment given to the patient and for all processes around the procedure (preparation and clearing up/ review).

Sources

Fintelmann V. *Intuitive Medizin. Einführung in eine anthroposophisch ergänzte Medizin.* Stuttgart: Hippokrates 1987.

Husemann F, Wolff O. *The Anthroposophical Approach to Medicine.* Vol. 1. Tr. P. Luborsky. Spring Valley: Anthroposophic Press 1982.

Kniebe G. *Die vier Elemente. Moderne Erfahrungen mit einer alten Wirklichkeit.* Stuttgart: Freies Geistesleben 1993.

Steiner R. *Theosophy.* Tr. C. E. Creeger. Hudson: Anthroposophic Press 1994.

Steiner R. *Anthroposophical Spiritual Science and Medical Therapy* (GA 313). Tr. rev. G. F. Karnow. Spring Valley: Mercury Press 1991.

Steiner R. *The Healing Process* (GA 319). Tr. C. E. Creeger. Hudson: Anthroposophic Press 2000.

Further reading

Husemann F, Wolff O. *Das Bild des Menschen als Grundlage der Heilkunst* Bd 2 und 3. Stuttgart: Freies Geistesleben 1991.

Steiner R, Wegman I. *Extending Practical Medicine* (GA 27). Tr. A. R. Meuss. London: Rudolf Steiner Press 1996.

3   Functional threefoldness in the human organism

Considering the way the human organism functions, we find basically there are three elementary processes at the different levels of cell, organ and organ system.

With the first group of processes it is a matter of the organism's ability to receive information (sensory impressions, stimuli, etc.) via the neurosensory system, process it and respond. The information has 'signal' character and does not take the form of physical matter.

The second group are metabolic by nature. In the metabolic system, substances are taken up into the organism, processed and eliminated again. The whole is highly dynamic and subject to continuous change and transformation. These processes are the polar opposite of those in the neurosensory system. 'Where information equals system and order, matter equals energy. Metabolism is therefore always the conversion of energy.' [Rohen 2000].

The third group of processes are rhythmical and hold a middle position between the information and metabolic processes. The latter two occur together in every organ and cell but are polar opposites and need to be brought into harmony. This happens through rhythm and periodicity. Organic life can only maintain itself by means of the rhythmical alternation between sleeping and waking, anabolism and catabolism, inhalation and exhalation, etc.

Each of the three processes is based on specific organic structures. Information processes have their centre in the neurosensory system, rhythmical processes in the cardiovascular and respiratory system and metabolic processes in the system of metabolism and limbs.

The three types of function in the human organism provide another approach in considering the phenomena of life in relation to human organic functions or processes. R. Steiner described them for the first time in 1917, in an appendix to his book *Von Seelenraetseln* [extracts in *The Case for Anthroposophy*]. He described the three types of

processes and then took this further by showing the relationship between them and the fundamental powers of the human soul – thinking, feeling and will.

3.1   The neurosensory system

In the neurosensory system we again find three different kinds of processes with their relevant organic structures. Sense organs take in the information, which is then processed in the brain. Nerve fibres and end organs serve to respond to stimuli, ultimately leading to neural control of all biological processes.

The central area, which is concentrated in the head, provides the physical basis for our everyday state of consciousness. The processes in the peripheral neural plexuses do not come to conscious awareness.

Specific principles in all three functional systems characterize the systems and are essential for healthy function. The principles which apply in the neurosensory system are well illustrated in the photograph of snow crystals (see over) – rest, coolness and a rich variety of forms that show distinct symmetry.

3.1.1   Principles

The principle of being at rest
This is well demonstrated by the brain itself which rests within the bony structures of the skull, enclosed in its spherical form. It is made weightless by the cerebrospinal fluid. As soon as the restful state is upset, e.g. due to concussion, brain function and the general state of well-being are seriously affected, as is general mobility.

The principle of coolness
Compared to other organ systems, the temperature in the brain is somewhat 'below normal'. The temperature of blood coming up from the metabolic sphere in the inferior vena cava,

for instance, is between 1.4 and 1.6 °C higher than the blood in the superior vena cava which comes from the head region (Husemann/Wolff – see Sources above). If the coolness has to give way to increased metabolic activity as in the case of a fever, the head responds relatively quickly with a headache, it gets difficult to concentrate and there may even be reduced consciousness or unconsciousness.

The principle of symmetry

The symmetrical configuration of the brain and the spinal cord with its rhythmical order is striking. This mirror-image arrangement of structures is, among other things, an important precondition for processes of conscious awareness in the neurosensory system.

The three principles, which we have only touched on, give us a picture for the morphology and function of the neurosensory system. They characterize the resting and structuring 'form pole' of the human organism.

3.1.2   Soul and spirit

The neurosensory system provides the bodily basis on which we are able to develop full consciousness and form ideas. As already mentioned, (immaterial) information in the form of sensory perceptions is received by this system and processed in thought; the end organs then respond to this. This gives us a real image of ourselves and the world, and we are able to gain insight into and explore the world, gaining orientation in it.

3.1.3   Catabolic processes

The functions of the neurosensory system result in destructive processes in the organism that may show themselves as tiredness by the end of a day or after a meeting that called for concentration. These processes are due to increased astral-body activity in the system as it transforms the constructive powers of the ether body into conscious awareness (see Basic principles, 2.7).

If the destructive processes overwhelm the constructive powers (of metabolism and limbs) for an extended period of time, this results in hardening and ultimately rigidity. The situation may arise in any organ system. Many of the signs of old age that go hand in hand with hardening and rigidity (e.g. chronic osteoarthritis) can be seen to be due to these processes.

3.2   The system of metabolism and limbs

The polar opposite to the neurosensory system is that of metabolism and limbs. We find its processes, too, in every organ and cell. They involve the intake of substances, their conversion into energies and final elimination. The organs enclosed by the peritoneum in the abdominal cavity are representative of the system. In the widest sense, the kidneys, too, may be included as an important eliminatory organ.

Different principles apply in this system, for it

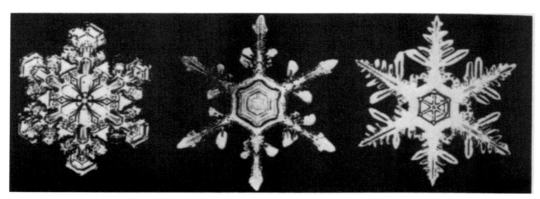

Fig. 1.3   Snow crystals (from Kniebe G. *Die vier Elemente*. Stuttgart: Freies Geistesleben 1993).

lives wholly in change and transformation. The image of a flame encompasses all the principles characteristic of this system — movement, the generation of heat, and asymmetry.

3.2.1   Principles

Mobility
Both in the digestive tract, at the centre of the system, and in the muscular system, all is continuous movement and dynamics, with matter taken up, transformed and changed into energy, exchanged and eliminated. Pathological conditions develop as soon as a state of rest occurs in the system, e.g. in the form of ileus.

Generation of warmth
A characteristic feature of activities in metabolism and limbs is the connection with warmth processes in the evolution and conversion of energies. This is due to marked ether-body activity in this system. The I-organization differentiates the generated warmth for the different organ systems. It can only do so, however, because limbs and metabolism first make the warmth available.

Asymmetry
Many of the organs that serve metabolism are asymmetrical — liver, stomach, intestine and pancreas. This system is the polar opposite of the neurosensory system which is highly differentiated and governed by symmetry. As already mentioned, symmetry has to do with the potential for conscious awareness. The unconscious processes in the system of metabolism and limbs show a correspondingly asymmetrical configuration.

3.2.2   Soul and spirit

Where the neurosensory system receives information from sensory perception and processes it in thought, the system of limbs and metabolism deals with substances from the world (substance pole). This provides the basis for human beings to get involved in the world, actively using their limbs.

The system of metabolism and limbs thus provides the bodily basis for the human will. Unlike thought processes, these will processes are at an unconscious level and we are unable to bring them to full awareness.

3.2.3   Anabolic processes

Metabolic processes are vital and constructive (see Basic principles, 2.5). For as long as they occur at a suitable level, ether-body activity makes the generation of warmth, body maintenance, growth and regeneration possible in all parts of the organism. These processes serve to keep the organism in health.

Inflammatory processes occur when anabolism is excessive (*calor*, *rubor*, etc.). Fever is a classic symptom where a raised body temperature reflects excessive metabolism which also leads to impairment in the neurosensory sphere, with hypersensitivity, reduced powers of concentration, headaches, and perhaps even reduced or loss of consciousness.

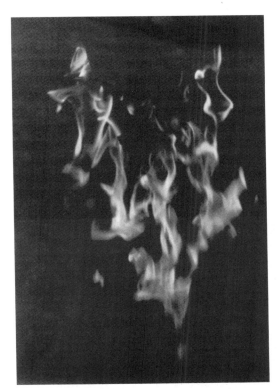

Fig. 1.4   Flame (from Kniebe G. *Die vier Elemente*. Stuttgart: Freies Geistesleben 1993).

The system of limbs and metabolism and the neurosensory system may thus be said to be playing opposite parts, with completely opposite functions and principles. If they were to impinge directly on one another, a state would develop that was wholly chaotic and not compatible with life, as the two systems would impede one another. Wise creator spirits have therefore developed a third system which mediates between these two.

3.3   The rhythmical system

Specifically rhythmical or periodical processes include the respiratory and circulatory functions. These, too, can be divided into three basic elements – intake of respiratory gases, 'conversion' of these in the lungs and body tissues, and elimination. Periodical processes may be discerned not only in the respiratory but also in the circulatory system which has distributing and transport functions. The heart is the central organ for this, ordering and distributing the blood streams and thus also regulating the functions in the capillaries.

The rhythmical processes are polar within themselves. In a way they practise their mediating function (form and substance poles) inwardly. This gives the rhythmical system the potential and justification for establishing and maintaining the right measure between the polar opposites. It thus serves the other two systems without regard for its own 'interests'.

The image of the wave illustrates the principles characteristic for the rhythmical system – polarity and creating a balance, constant renewal and flexible adaptation. (Plate, Figure 3)

3.3.1   Principles

The breathing rhythm is 'the' rhythmical process. It may serve as an example for elucidating the principles of rhythm.

The polarity and balance principle
On inhalation, the chest expands, air rich in oxygen flows into the expanding space in the lungs and oxygen exchange takes place in the blood. When the high point has been reached, the process reverses. On exhalation the chest contracts, air containing little oxygen is released to the outside, until the low point is reached and the process turned around again, with new air streaming in.

Every breath thus shows itself to be a polar process in which extremes arise and pass away again, balanced out in the process. It is the direction of the air flow which is polar, with the tension that has built up on inhalation released again on exhalation.

The 'constant renewal' principle
This beginning and ending of polarity and balance happens over and over again. The process is continually renewed. Unlike an engine, however, where processes are exactly the same as they repeat themselves, with no deviation in time, the 'repetitions' which occur in the sphere of life show minor variations.

Constant renewal thus means continuous repetition of something *similar*. Every breath, every heartbeat differs slightly from the one that went before. It may not be quite so strong, or a hundredth of a second faster or slower. These minor deviations are reviving and refreshing. Anything lacking in rhythm, anything rigid and immovable drains energy.

The 'flexible adaptation' principle
Rhythmical processes such as breathing and heartbeat adapt to demands coming from outside by changing their frequency. The heart will beat faster and our breathing will speed up when we climb stairs, for instance. As soon as

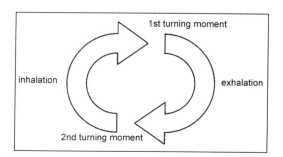

Fig. 1.5   Polarity in breathing.

the demands cease, the situation calms down again, returning to the base line.

3.3.2   Soul and spirit

The rhythmical system provides the bodily basis for the soul's ability to feel. It will correspondingly react to emotions (e.g. by accelerating our breathing or heartbeat). Feelings tend to develop at a dreamlike level of consciousness. Even when they are not coming to full awareness (e.g. in thinking activities) it is possible to become fully conscious of them by developing our own inner activity.

The powerful connection between physiological processes and the emotional life becomes very evident when there is organic disease. When threatening conditions arise due to respiratory or cardiac malfunction (e.g. in cases of asthma or myocardial infarction), intense fear of death is felt by the individual, and no external factor will relieve it. In these cases the emotional equilibrium is seriously upset due to organic disease, and healthy organic function has to be restored before harmony can return also to the emotional life.

3.3.3   Rhythm and health

We see rhythms in many natural phenomena such as the changing seasons, the tides, or night and day; in the onrush of the waves, or growth periods in the plant world — flower, fruit, withering. Rhythms are time phenomena in the sphere of life, a sequence of similar processes that continue to repeat themselves.

The way we see things today, rhythm belongs to the musical element which comes to expression in speech, dance, movement and music itself. Rhythm is a kind of spiritual order given to movement to help something which is of the essence to show itself in space and time. In this sense, rhythm mediates between spiritual realities (the essence or spirit) and things that are given on earth (phenomena). Rudolf Steiner therefore also considered rhythm to be semi-spiritual by nature.

We all know how valuable rhythm is for maintaining health in everyday life. We also know how lack of rhythm can affect our health when we have to work in shifts or at night. Rhythmically recurring activities help to restore health also in sickness, and nursing and therapies should therefore always be rhythmical. This alone will contribute to self healing and establish a healthy balance. The beneficial effect must be said to be mainly due to the fact that the rhythmical element brings spiritual qualities directly into the sphere of earthly life.

Health is thus seen to arise when the rhythmical system maintains a biological balance between the nourishing and regenerating (though unconscious) constructive processes in the system of metabolism and limbs on the one hand and the destructive processes of the neurosensory system (which do, however, provide the potential for conscious awareness). In this respect, the Einreibungen, being rhythmical, create harmony between these two opposite poles and thus strengthen the powers that keep the human organism in health. Table 1.2 sums up the three systems and their qualities.

Table 1.2 Functional threefoldness			
	Neurosensory system	Rhythmical system	Metabolism and limbs
Representative organ	brain and spinal marrow sense organs	heart lung	digestive organs muscles
Principles	rest coldness symmetry	polarity and balance constant renewal flexible adaptation	movement warmth asymmetry
Morbid tendency	sclerosis		inflammation
Conscious awareness	awake	dreaming	dim
Soul capacity	thinking	feeling	will, doing

3.4   Functional threefold qualities and Rhythmical Einreibungen

A Rhythmical Einreibung addresses all the areas known to us from the three functional spheres. The neurosensory sphere receives impulses mainly through direct skin contact and the use of fragrant substances (see Part 4). The metabolic sphere is also stimulated, as evident from the warmth generated and increased blood flow.

The rhythmical element of the treatment presents an ideal to the patient's rhythmical system so that this may get a clearer picture again of its function as a mediator between the two opposites.

It therefore has to be realized that irrespective of the area treated, every Rhythmical Einreibung has an effect on all rhythmical processes. The breathing grows calmer and deeper, the sleep-waking rhythm grows more regular, and digestive functions are stimulated. The treatments are therefore an instrument we use to address the whole human being and in particular the powers that maintain health.

Properly thought-out and targeted use of Rhythmical Einreibungen first of all calls for a diagnosis of the relationship between functional processes. This will provide general pointers to the choice of method. When neurosensory processes predominate, we choose a treatment that will support the metabolic processes. The technique chosen will be warming, loosening and dynamic. When metabolic processes predominate, we choose a treatment with calm, structure and clarity to strengthen the neurosensory pole, thus helping to restore a harmonious balance.

Sources
Fintelmann V. *Intuitive Medizin. Einführung in eine anthroposophisch ergaenzte Medizin.* Stuttgart: Hippokrates 1987.

Hoerner W. *Zeit und Rhythmus. Die Ordnungsgesetze der Erde und des Menschen.* 2. Aufl. Stuttgart: Urachhaus 1991.

Rohen JW. *Morphologie des menschlichen Organimus.* Stuttgart: Freies Geistesleben 2000.

Steiner R. *Von Seelenraetseln* (GA 21). 5. Aufl. Dornach: Rudolf Steiner-Nachlassverwaltung 1983. Extracts in *The Case for Anthroposophy.* Tr. O. Barfield. London: Rudolf Steiner Press 1970.

Steiner R. *Anthroposophical Spiritual Science and Medical Therapy* (GA 313). Tr. rev. G. F. Karnow. Spring Valley: Mercury Press 1991.

Steiner R. *The Healing Process* (GA 319). Tr. C. E. Creeger. Hudson: Anthroposophic Press 2000.

Further reading
Buehler W. *Der Leib als Instrument der Seele.* 8. Aufl. Stuttgart: Freies Geistesleben 1981.

4   The senses

From the anthroposophical point of view, there are twelve spheres of sensory perception. These provide for comprehensive perception of one's own body, the surrounding world and other human beings. Studying the twelve senses, nurses can gain ideas for the work they do for and with patients, extending the range of their professional expertise.

Rhythmical Einreibungen specifically address the human being as a life form capable of sensory perception. They convey a vast abundance of (sensory) experiences which have a direct influence on the individual's physical and mental well-being.

Feelings and thoughts follow a patient's sensory perceptions, for these provoke inner responses and want to be understood.

Distinction is made between processes of

1   sensory perception. The sense organ takes in sensations of colour, smell or warmth, for instance. Information on the outside world thus enters into the person's inner life.
2   inner experience. The individual reacts emotionally to the 'information' received via a sense organ. This process and sensory perception generally take place without the conscious mind being involved. For as long as our sense organs are sound and opportunities for sensory perception arise, they will always be ready to take in more. The inner response follows immediately, irrespective of whether the sensory impressions come to conscious awareness or not.
3   insight and understanding. We think about the perceptions made and integrate them in our fund of knowledge. This process does not automatically follow sensory perception and inner response, for it needs the human I to enter into an active thought process. In giving the Rhythmical Einreibungen we always address the I of the individual in every process of gaining insight that arises.

We are deliberately not going into the epistemological background, as it would take us too

far and does not relate directly to the present subject. Reference will, however, be made to further reading.

Both humans and animals have sense organs which are part of and enrich the inner life of the soul. Unlike the animals, human beings are not forced, however, to react to their perceptions from pure instinct. Instead, a rational mind and common sense allow them to deal with the reactions and the insights they have gained at the level of body, soul or spirit. Humans are therefore freer, able to make choices, when it comes to their responses to sensory perceptions. Animals cannot influence their reactions at will.

4.1   The twelve senses

If we consider elements which different senses have in common, we arrive at three groups of four – senses relating to body, soul and spirit. Every sense has its own organ and this mediates specific sensory perceptions. In the anthroposophical literature, Rudolf Steiner and other authors refer to physical organs also for senses that are not known in conventional science. These are mentioned here for the sake of completeness but not considered in detail.

We use the first four senses, also known as the 'bodily senses' to perceive our own body. The next four enable us to perceive the world around us. They particularly evoke feelings in us, which is why they are also called the 'senses of feeling or of the soul'. The third group of senses enables us to perceive spiritual aspects specifically with reference to human beings. They are therefore also called the 'spiritual senses'.

The twelve senses enable us to experience the whole of ourselves and the world around us. Although we are able to perceive these qualities with 'normal' senses, they do reflect twelve different spiritual powers of configuration in the cosmos [H. E. Lauer. *Die 12 Sinne des Men-*

schen, 1977]. The qualities perceived give us inner experiences that affect the psyche even when we are not always fully aware of this. The kind of sensory impressions to which we expose ourselves do make a difference, for our choice does affect the mood of soul.

In the description of the senses which follows, the emphasis is on the senses which are particularly significant in the context of Rhythmical Einreibungen. These are the bodily senses, the sense of smell and the sense of warmth.

4.1.1   Sense of touch

Touch sensations are highly complex, being made up of impressions gained in the sensory perceptions of touch, life, one's own movement, balance and warmth. They also arise with sensory activities other than the touching of an object. Thus the eye scans the outside world when we are looking for something, the tongue uses touch when tasting, and the sense of hearing feels its way through space when we listen. Memories and judgements are part of the process when we use touch, as with all sensory impressions. It is, however, possible to be quite specific about a field of sensory perception that is entirely touch and about the inner experiences which are connected with this.

This is really perception of one's own body. We perceive the effects which an outside object has on the body. Judgement as to whether an object is hard or soft depends on the effort needed to effect a change in the object. This is considerable if the object is hard, and slight if it is soft. We thus experience the resistance offered by the object we touch. There is something of a paradox in this. We hope that feeling our way by touch will take us into the outside world, yet all we experience is our own body.

We thus experience our own boundaries in space. Yet although we ultimately cannot go beyond these, touch does convey a feeling of inner certainty and security as we learn about our outer boundaries. People who no longer have a sense of touch will react with feelings of anxiety. This kind of anxiety reflects a general state of mind induced by loss of inner certainty.

The situation exists with patients who have been bedridden for a long time; it is even greater in the field of intensive care. Seriously ill

Table 1.3 The twelve senses		
Sense	Sensory perception	Sense organ
Bodily senses of		
1 touch	feel by touch	tactile corpuscles in the skin
2 life	subjective feeling in body	autonomic nervous system
3 (own) movement	own motion	muscle and tendon spindles
4 balance	orientation in space	organ of balance
Senses of feeling or the soul		
5 smell	odour	olfactory epithelium in the nose
6 taste	taste	taste buds in the tongue
7 sight or vision	colours	eye
8 warmth	relationship between own and ambient warmth	temperature receptors in the skin
Spiritual senses		
9 hearing	sounds, noises	ear
10 sound or word	speech sounds (vowels, consonants)	physical organism of capacity for movement
11 thought or concept	thoughts, concepts	physical organism of the whole body
12 I	the I of another (you)	whole physical sensory configuration of the human being

patients are prophylactically positioned in a way that conveys a kind of weightlessness. Patients find this a real trauma, for they can no longer sense their own body and lose that elementary feeling of inner certainty.

Through touch, a Rhythmical Einreibung can therefore strengthen the individual's feeling of inner certainty, reducing fear and anxiety.

4.1.2   Sense of life

This sense is not part of the general physiology of the senses. Rudolf Steiner described it as a sense which, in a way, reflects the functioning of our vital processes. We may use the analogy of a lake and the way the sky is reflected in its surface. Meadows and hills surrounding the lake give it its own character. Yet every lake, be it in the mountains or in the plains, reflects the part of the sky which is above it. In a similar way we have the sense of life as a reflector for the inner aspect of our vital processes.

The actual experience of the sense of life is a feeling of being at ease, at home in one's own body for as long as the vital processes are in harmony. We do not perceive the vital processes as such, therefore, but the feelings of ease connected with them.

It is on the basis of these that the human being feels himself to be at home in his earthly existence. If that sense of well-being is upset and malaise, tiredness or even sensations of being ill develop, this feeling of 'being at home' will also be lost. We then leave the sense of life's sphere of perception as we become aware of sensations in individual organs. These come to conscious awareness by a different route than by the sense of life [K. Koenig].

4.1.3   Sense of one's own movement

This is another sense in the group of four which serve to convey a feeling to us for the condition of our own body, thus providing a living sense of our bodily existence.

The sense of our own movement allows us to perceive the position, attitude and relative position of the parts of our body. We are thus able at any time to be aware of the position of a hand, for example, our posture, or the movements of arms and legs. We perceive where the parts of the body are and how they relate to one another. The precondition is that the body is in motion. In that case we do on the one hand perceive the relative positions of our body parts and are on the other hand able to coordinate their movement for a given purpose, getting the movement to be meaningful and fluid.

Young children in particular show us that perception of one's own movement gives a feeling of joy. The perceptions of this sense enable us to feel ourselves as free human beings as we move and to take pleasure in this.

During Rhythmical Einreibungen, this perception is perhaps less significant than the experiences gained through the senses of touch and life, for their own movements are always less important to those who are receiving the treatment. Their limbs tend to be at rest. They move only when we change the positioning of a patient.

On the other hand the sense of one's own movement is more involved in perceiving the different forms of the treatment. According to Rudolf Steiner, this sense is also involved when we recreate the form of a circle with our eyes, for example. It thus serves not only to perceive the movements made by our own body, but also mediates living experience of form and movement tendencies in the world around us. The different basic forms of the Rhythmical Einreibungen therefore lead to a living experience which is connected with the character of these forms.

4.1.4   Sense of balance

This sense enables us to experience the dimensions in space and find our place within them. Above/below, left/right, in front/behind give us our orientation in space. This applies to our own bodies as well as the location of touch, visual and acoustic impressions. Perceptions made through the sense of balance thus also accompany other sensory impressions (seeing, hearing).

The perceptions gained through the sense of

balance let human beings know themselves to be existing independently of space and time. Out of an inner calm, an inner equilibrium, they find that they do not change when moving in space, staying the same and taking themselves in their body to wherever they go, independent of space.

Although the treatments are largely done with the patients lying down, the direction given to the forms does convey a sense of their own uprightness, of front and back, left and right.

We are leaving the sphere of bodily senses with the sense of balance, and now turn to the 'senses of feeling'. With regard to the Rhythmical Einreibungen, particular significance attaches to the senses of smell and of warmth.

4.1.5   Sense of smell

Smells can only be perceived via the airy element. We perceive inner qualities of the body from which the scent or smell comes.

Intense emotional reactions relate to the smells we perceive. They may range from utter disgust to wanting to give ourselves wholly to an aroma. Smells will often call up memories of situations we have known in life. Thus the smell of newly ground grain may recall cornfields on a summer holiday, or a scent of cinnamon and other spices may take us back to childhood Christmases. In such situations our memories are particularly coloured by the feelings that go with them.

It is difficult if not impossible to distance yourself inwardly from smells, for the sensation of smell is physiologically linked with the process of inhalation. In this respect we are actually forced all the time to take into ourselves the particular part of the world the qualities of which are perceived through the sense of smell.

Aromatherapy is based on the use of specific scents. This bears out the importance of perceptions of smell. The scent of substances used with Rhythmical Einreibungen therefore has a role to play. The comforting, harmonizing or stimulating effects of the treatments can be emphasized and strengthened by it.

4.1.6   Sense of taste

Tastes can only be perceived via the watery element. Foods must be chewed and mixed with saliva (watered down) in the mouth before we experience the four taste qualities of sweet, salty, sour and bitter.

Like smell, taste tells us something about a specific condition of a body. It makes a big difference with regard to taste if a plant has produced sugars or bitter compounds, for instance, and at the same time also tells us something about different developmental processes in plants [W. Pelikan].

Like the sense of smell, the sense of taste relates closely to our feelings. The reaction to a particular taste will depend on our personal 'taste'. Generally speaking we may say that sweet tastes tend to please us, whilst bitter tastes are considered more unpleasant.

4.1.7   Sense of vision

The term 'to perceive' is often equated with 'to see', which makes us aware of the dominance of this sense.

We only perceive coloured surfaces and degrees of shade. A complex thought process makes us identify the surfaces perceived to be a tree or a church. Thus we do not, in fact, see a lake but a blue surface surrounded by, let us say, a green one. When we then identify this blue surface area as a lake set in grassland we have come to this conclusion on the basis of various processes of remembering and forming an opinion.

The inner experiences connected with visual perception are many and varied, for vision lets us perceive the world of colours and above all gain knowledge of the world around us. We also develop quite specific emotional reactions in connection with the experience of colour. Thus green is calming, whereas red rouses us to activity.

4.1.8   Sense of warmth

The sense of warmth serves to perceive the difference in temperature between an object and our own body. The information is therefore not absolute but relative.

Warmth and coldness (absence of warmth) evoke marked emotional reactions. People have individual standards, preferences and dislikes in this respect, depending on the nature of their own warmth organism.

Rhythmical Einreibungen are intended to address also the human warmth organism. The perception of warmth therefore plays a major role during the treatment. This begins with taking note of the room temperature before and after treatment, and goes all the way to the temperature of the carers' hands. As soon as the room or the hands are too cold – cold tending to be more of a problem than warmth – we have unfavourable conditions for effective treatment. Patients also tend to show shock reactions or simply do not feel well when touched with cold hands or if they feel cold during a treatment. Special care must therefore be taken in creating the right warmth conditions.

The next four senses mainly perceive the spiritual in human beings. They are not addressed directly when Rhythmical Einreibungen are given, but are nevertheless involved. With the exception of the sense of hearing these senses are not formally known in conventional medicine. It therefore also needs some practice and insight before one is able to work consciously with these senses and the spheres of sensory perception relating to them.

4.1.9   Sense of hearing

The perception of sounds and noises is made possible by the sense of hearing. We perceive the 'inwardness' of an entity. An object begins to sound when it is made to vibrate – a bell, for example. The sound tells us something of its inmost nature. This applies particularly to the human voice, for every human voice has its characteristic tone. It has a musical quality.

4.1.10   Sense of word or sound

To experience this sense on its own it may be helpful to think of the sound of a foreign language – Japanese perhaps, or Arabic – and ask yourself: What do these sounds/this melody of speech tell me? How does someone learn to think and find inner responses who grows up with this as his mother tongue?

Sounds (vowels or consonants) have a quality of their own, independent of the meaning of a word, and this is perceived through the sense of sound (tone).

It is difficult to distinguish between the sound and meaning of a word and we are not in the habit of doing so, for we focus on the meaning of a word as soon as we hear it. The whole is a complex process of sensory perception. We hear a melody of speech (sound) and perceive the meaning of what has been said (concept). Thinking often follows, taking hold of the perception and gaining full understanding.

In eurythmy, an art form developed by Rudolf Steiner, sounds are made visible in gesture and movement. Every sound of the alphabet has its own character and this is carefully worked out and made 'visible'. Seeing eurythmy performed or doing it oneself is thus another way of coming closer to the inherent quality of speech sounds.

4.1.11   Sense of thought

With this sense, human beings are able to perceive a thought or idea conveyed in speech sounds. Distinction is therefore made between words (speech) and the meaning of words (concepts).

Thus it is possible, for instance, to communicate without words in a country where one does not know the language. We then tend to use not only speech but also hands and feet (gesture) to express ourselves, and after a time it is generally possible to communicate in this way. Knowledge of the language is less important in this case than perceiving the meaning of what the other person wants to communicate. The other person's thought is taken in through words and also gestures.

4.1.12   Sense of self or I

This sense allows us to perceive the individual nature or personality of another person and not our own self, as might be assumed.

The most important part of perceiving another I is to find the other person to be different from oneself. The process of perception lies in the interplay between 'perceiving the other' and 'coming to yourself'. Moving to and fro between 'you' and 'me' lets us perceive the individual nature of the other. This also involves perceptions made with all the other senses – a precondition for the sense of self or I.

4.2   The twelve senses and Rhythmical Einreibungen

Perceptions made with the bodily senses always involve all of them. This wholeness makes us feel ourselves to be a complete organism in the space that surrounds us. We come to terms with our bodily nature and its boundaries in relation to the outside, thus establishing the 'I and world' relationship. With Rhythmical Einreibungen, applied in direct contact with the body and therefore moving essentially though not exclusively in the sphere of perception that belongs to these senses, the patient receives elementary experiences of the body and important inner experiences connected with this. In a very intimate way, awareness is created for qualities which people tend to have lost in the case of sickness. Above all they are given an image of their own body that puts them at ease, where before the whole or areas of it were felt to be difficult and an impediment. They are able to feel 'at home' again, at least for a time, in 'their own four walls', and to make their peace with their own body.

Using the middle senses, people take in knowledge or qualities of the surrounding world. The inner experiences which arise in the process are highly emotive by nature. Working consciously with the perceptive qualities of these senses we are thus able to address specifically the individual's life of feeling. In nursing, this may be done by selecting suitable aromatic substances, well-seasoned meals, a good choice of colours for the sickroom to create harmony, or putting paintings or prints on the walls of corridors and rooms. The choice of substance for a treatment allows specific aromatic qualities to be brought in. Being careful about warmth (for the patient and of our hands) will do the patient good. It is part of the elementary basis of the treatment.

The sound, word, thought and I of the other person convey something of his or her nature. These perceptions may not always be consciously considered in the nursing procedure but they exist and have a major influence on the nurse-patient relationship. Many patients are particularly wide-awake in this sphere of the senses, taking in a great deal of the carer's individual nature. Conversely, carers may learn a lot about their patients and take it into account in their work. It is worthwhile, therefore, to be conscious of the way we speak, to cultivate the life of our thoughts, and to be fully present in mind as we make contact with another individual.

Sources
Koenig K. *Sinnesentwicklung und Leiberfahrung*. 3. Aufl. Stuttgart: Freies Geistesleben 1986. *The Human Soul*. Edinburgh: Floris.
Lehrs E. *Vom Geist der Sinne*. 2. Aufl. Frankfurt 1982.
Lindenberg C (ed.). *Zur Sinneslehre. Rudolf Steiner. Themen aus dem Gesamtwerk* Band 3. Stuttgart: Freies Geistesleben.
Pelikan W. *Healing Plants* (vol. 1 of his botany of medicinal plants). Tr. A. Meuss. Spring Valley: Mercury Press 1997.
Rohen JW. *Morphologie des menschlichen Organismus*. Stuttgart: Freies Geistesleben 2000.
Steiner R. *Anthroposophy – a Fragment* (GA 45). Tr. C.E. Creeger, D. Hardorp. New York: Anthroposophic Press 1996.
Steiner R. *A Psychology of Body, Soul and Spirit* (GA 115). Tr. M. Spock. Hudson: Anthroposophic Press 1999.
Steiner R. *The Philosophy of Freedom. A Philosophy of Spiritual Activity* (GA 4). Tr. R. Stebbing. London: Rudolf Steiner Press 1988. Also as *Intuitive Thinking as a Spiritual Path*. Tr. M. Lipson. Hudson: Anthroposophic Press 1995.
Steiner R. *Conferences with the Teachers of the Waldorf School in Stuttgart* vol. 1 (GA 300a). Tr. P. Wehrle. Sussex: Steiner Schools Fellowship 1986. Also as *Faculty Meetings with Rudolf Steiner*. Tr. W. Lathe, N.P. Whittaker. Hudson: Anthroposophic Press 1998.

Further reading

Sayre-Adams J, Wright S. *Therapeutische Beruehrung in Theorie und Praxis*. Berlin: Ullstein Mosby 1997.

Steiner R. *The Science of Knowing* (GA 2). Tr. W. Lindeman. Spring Valley: Mercury Press 1988.

Steiner R. *Truth and Science* (GA 3). Tr. W. Lindeman. Spring Valley: Mercury Press.

Steiner R. *The Riddle of Humanity* (GA 170). Tr. J. F. Logan. London: Rudolf Steiner Press 1990.

Steiner R. *The Study of Man* (GA 293). Tr. D. Harwood, H. Fox. London: Rudolf Steiner Publishing Co./Anthroposophic Press 1947. Also as *The Foundations of Human Experience*. Tr. R.F. Lathe, N. Parsons Whittaker, H. Barnes. Hudson: Anthroposophic Press 1996.

Steiner R. *From Comets to Cocaine* GA 348). Answers to Questions. Tr. M. St Goar, rev. M. Barton. London: Rudolf Steiner Press 2000. Also as *Health and Illness* vols 1 & 2. Tr. M. St Goar. New York: Anthroposophic Press.

Koenig K. *Der kreis der zwölf Sinne und die sieben Lebensprozesse*. Stuttgart: Freies Geistesleben 1999.

5   The hand

The hand holds a special position in the organism. It enables us to take deliberate, creative action in the world. Hand and foot stand for something specifically human that is connected with our life on earth and the activities that shape the world.

Dr Margarethe Hauschka, who helped to develop the Rhythmical Einreibungen, described the hand as an organ that is wholly typical of the human being and his means of expressing himself:

'In the hand, finally, this finely modelled and organized member with its incredible potential for movement, the human spirit has created an instrument for itself that enables it to recreate any form in the realm of the form-giving powers – powers the ether body uses – and indeed to go beyond nature to build a new world, the world of the arts out of the substances of the earth. ... This characterizes the hand as the most human organ, for its physiognomy permits us to learn much of the human being's inmost nature. Gestures in particular, the way in which we shake hands, for instance, and much else, including involuntary movements, tell more about our character than we often like the world to know.' [1984]

Nursing is 'hands-on' work, and the hand is our most important instrument. We probably use it more frequently than anything else in nursing as we touch and treat another person. Working with the Rhythmical Einreibungen, carers can train their hands' powers of perception and expression, cultivating and perfecting these to serve the powers that restore health.

5.1.   The threefold hand

The human skeleton shows two tendencies which are polar opposites. The head region shows a round, spherical form principle. Bony plates predominate that enclose the skull cavity from outside. In the limbs, the situation is exactly the opposite, with tubular long bones

and joints lying between them, which makes the limbs extraordinarily mobile. Between these two extremes lies the trunk. It shows marked segmentation. Rhythmical repetition of similar elements such as vertebrae or ribs is the dominant form principle in this case.

The arms are connected with the middle region, the trunk, through the shoulder girdle. They, too, are in three sections (upper arm, forearm and hand). The forearm with its two bones and the articular joints allows many different hand positions ranging from supination to pronation. The number of bony elements and joints increases towards the periphery. In accordance with this, the potential for movement and expression of the upper limbs also increases in the direction of the hand.

Arms and hands are freely mobile. In their normal position they do not touch the ground (like the feet), nor do they point upwards. Their sphere of action is in the horizontal, though they are also capable of digging deep or reaching up high.

The threefold configuration makes the hand an organ for the expression and perception of human intentions. This makes it ideal for Rhythmical Einreibungen. The range of possible functions is reflected in the morphology and type of functions belonging to the three regions of the hand.

5.1.1   The neurosensory pole

The five fingers ('finger hand') are the neurosensory pole. Here the emphasis is on sensory perception and conscious awareness.

The phalanges are rays made up of long bones and a relatively large number of joints between them. The pad of the finger is highly sensitive to touch. The pointwise local touch typical of the fingertips will above all create conscious awareness when someone is touched in this way. This kind of touch awakens rather than letting us dream.

Such a waking state may be welcome in some

situations but not with Rhythmical Einreibungen. We therefore endeavour to counteract the point quality of the finger hand, giving it the touch quality of a plane.

5.1.2   The metabolic pole

Compared to the phalanges, the carpal bones are small and variable in shape. Unlike the finger part of the hand, where tendons predominate, the heel of the hand is furnished with more muscle in the thenar and hypothenar eminences. The metabolic and warmth processes of the hand are thus more concentrated in this area.

The function of the heel of the hand also shows an emphasis on the will element. Activities such as kneading dough are done with this part of the hand. We prop ourselves up on it and use it for pushing and exerting pressure. These activities reflect will impulses which often involve considerable strength. Perceptive capacity is, however, greatly reduced here.

The tendency is to press quite hard with this part of the hand when giving a treatment. The quality of the will element then predominates, and we leave the rhythmical sphere.

5.1.3   The rhythmical region

The metacarpus includes both poles, but in reduced form. The radial quality of the fingers has become a plane, with small muscle pads at the basal joints. Its mobility allows contact to be close, enveloping and pulsating. Warmth radiates to the whole hand from here.

Opening and closing movement starts from the middle part of the hand. Enveloping, receiving, warming and holding are specific functions for this part. The encounter between two people who shake hands also lies here. The middle part of the hand thus plays a particular role in contact between people.

Both perceptive and will-related qualities are found in this part of the hand, which gives it a special relationship to the rhythmical system. Its qualities come into play in giving form to a treatment.

Apart from distinguishing three regions of the hand, we can also see a fundamental difference in quality between the dorsum and the palm of the hand. The dorsum is more neuro-sensory by nature, whilst the palm has more of an emphasis on metabolism. This does not play a role in Rhythmical Einreibungen, as they are always given using the inside of the hand.

5.2   The hand as mediator

5.2.1   Touch

Touch opens up a world of impressions and events for us. The capacity for touch is the natural gift of every human being. In the light of our knowledge of the twelve senses we may see it as a comprehensive encounter between two individuals that happens not only on the physical level but also on those of soul and spirit.

In nursing, hands-on contact plays a special role, being part of many nursing interventions. Nurses are indisputably 'touchers by profession'. The degree to which physical contact is conscious or cultivated depends on the natural abilities of nurses and their professional development.

With this physical contact, patients learn something about the intentions and attitude of their nurse. They may sense kindness, indifference, empathy or encouragement. The quality and the care taken over physical contact are thus of vital importance to them. Rhythmical Einreibungen also involve intensive physical contact. Ideally they are done in a way that leaves both patient and nurse free, being neither oppressive nor noncommittal.

5.2.2   Straight line and circle

Apart from the experiences connected with the rhythmical element and the carer's intentions, patients also perceive the quality of form in a Rhythmical Einreibung. Forms are made up of two basic elements in many different variations – *straight line* and *circle*. What do we experience in looking at these forms? What inner experiences arise with them?

Table 1.4	
Straight Line	Circle
Straight	Curved
Gives structure	Enfolding
Cool	Warm
Separating right and left	Forming inner and outer space

Some of the many possible qualities experienced are shown in Table 1.4, which may help readers to develop a feeling for them.

The different qualities of the forms reflect fundamental elements in human and cosmic evolution that are either structural and hardening or dissolving and evanescent. In all spheres of life, processes move between these two extremes of solidification (neurosensory system) and dissolution (metabolism and limbs).

Hardening tendencies are particularly marked in the human skeletal system. Dissolving tendencies take the form of cell lysis, among other things. Degenerative joint disease and concretions thus reflect hardening processes, whilst infectious diseases or inflammatory changes involving a temperature show marked tendencies to dissolve. In the same way, moods may vary between the extremes of obstinacy and depression on the one hand and manic inconsistency or lack of responsibility on the other. In social and political life, these tendencies may range from oppressive dictatorship to lawless anarchy. The list of possible examples is endless.

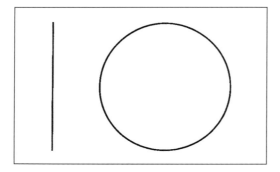

Fig. 1.6   Straight line and circle.

Both tendencies have their justification and are meaningful if they come at the right time and in the right place. They are destructive when the individual is not handling them with due care or if they go too much to an extreme. It is therefore important for every individual to establish the right balance between them in the conduct of life.

5.2.3   Circle and straight line in Rhythmical Einreibungen

With Rhythmical Einreibungen, we have these tendencies in the geometrical forms of circle and straight line. They are connected with specific effects, and this goes back to the hardening and dissolving processes. In most cases the circle dominates, for the aim is to give life and warmth to the tissues. In some instances it is, however, important to bring in a structuring element by using straight lines, and this is whenever there is too much mobility or warmth. It is always the patient's subjective well-being which governs our choice of emphasis, with careful observation of the processes or the phenomena that indicate them.

The rhythmical quality of the treatments means that every movement includes the polar opposites of straight line and curve. Increasing intensity, like systole or inhalation, has more the quality of the straight line – structured, cool, tensed, awakening and going all the way to closeness, anxiety and shock. Dissolution, or letting go, which has the same character as diastole or exhalation, relates more to roundedness – lying, warming, enveloping, relaxing to the point of dreaminess or sleep.

The straight or round element tends to predominate in a body region, depending on its character. With Rhythmical Einreibungen, alternation between increasing intensity and letting go balances out the polar extremes with every stroke, circle and spiral movement.

It is also possible to increase the straight element and so give direction and structure where metabolism is overweening (strokes down the back), or to give emphasis to the rounded element with its specially warming quality to counteract coolness, rigidity or stiffness (arthritis of the knee).

Sources

Hauschka M. *Rhythmical Massage as Indicated by Ita Wegman*. London: Rudolf Steiner Press 1979.

Rohen JW. *Morphologie des menschlichen Organimus*. Stuttgart: Freies Geistesleben 2000.

Steiner R. Die *Polaritaet von Dauer und Entwickelung im Menschenleben* (GA 184). 2. Aufl. Dornach: Rudolf Steiner Nachlassverwaltung 1983. Six of the lectures in English in *Three Streams in the Evolution of Mankind*. Tr. C. Davy. London: Rudolf Steiner Press 1965.

Further reading

Grossmann-Schnyder M. *Beruehren. Praktischer Leitfaden zur Psychotonik in Pflege und Therapie*. 3. Aufl. Stuttgart: Hippokrates 2000.

Husemann AJ. *The Harmony of the Human Body*. Tr. C. von Arnim. Edinburgh: Floris Books 1994.

Montague A. *Koerperkontakt*. 7. Aufl. Klett-Cotta, Stuttgart 1992.

Sayre-Adams H, Wright S. *Therapeutische Beruehrung in Theorie und Praxis*. Berlin: Ullstein Mosby 1997.

Chapter 2
Quality criteria for Rhythmical Einreibungen according to Wegman/Hauschka

Edelgard Grosse-Brauckmann

Writing these pages I found once again that giving thought to the subject brings not only further clarification but also new questions. Readers are therefore asked to take this not as something complete and fully matured but as something about which we may enter into dialogue.

At this point I wish to express my gratitude to everyone who contributed to these pages as they now are by reading the proofs and discussing them with me.

1   Introduction

Nurses are 'touchers by profession'. Until the turn of the 20th century it was taken for granted that they had a natural gift for this, and until a few decades ago 'physical contact' was not part of the training school curriculum.

The situation has changed a great deal since then. Ideas, techniques and disciplines have developed where physical contact ranks high. Examples are the Alexander Technique, acupressure, aromatherapy, chirophonetics, craniosacral therapy, osteopathy and therapeutic touch. All of them have to do with the connection which exists between body, soul and spirit and the knowledge that self-healing powers can be stimulated without resorting to medicinal agents. This also involves using your hands to help people and finding ways of developing your natural ability further.

Carers interested in nursing care extended through anthroposophy came to ask themselves: How can additional points of view and practical suggestions for professional physical contact be found through anthroposophy? It meant adding something to the things that were already being done in nursing. Their thinking was governed by the question as to the nature of a truly human touch and how this might be brought into play. Dr Ita Wegman had developed the method of Rhythmical Massage and this seemed to be an area where one might look for what was needed in nursing. Ultimately the search led to the Rhythmical Einreibungen according to Wegman/Hauschka.

These have now been practised by many carers around the world for about 80 years. The method is not strictly defined, as both the practice and the teaching of it demand continuous further development. In future, closer collaboration with scientists investigating rhythms and the nursing sciences is bound to bear fruit in our search for insight into, and our use of, Rhythmical Einreibungen.

Some of the above-mentioned contact therapies are now so much part of nursing that we also cannot imagine doing without them in anthroposophical clinics and hospitals. In the following pages, the attempt is made to show 1) the value of Rhythmical Einreibungen, 2) where the emphasis lies with them, and 3) how they can complement other methods.

2   The origins of Rhythmical Einreibungen

Rhythmical Einreibungen have been developed from Rhythmical Massage Therapy according to Wegman/Hauschka. Let us consider some characteristics of Rhythmical Massage Therapy before we come to the connection between Rhythmical Einreibungen and Rhythmical Massage Therapy. The latter is a development of classic massage, extending it on the basis of the anthroposophical view of the human being. It addresses the organization which supports life in the human being – the life body – and the higher bodies known as the soul and the I-organization.

This is brought to realization in specific techniques and in the range of effects and possible uses. All techniques (effleurage, airy kneading, friction, vibration, percussion) are characteristically *light*, i.e. *no physical pressure* is exerted by the hands. We speak of 'suction' or 'negative pressure' here.

The carer's posture is wholly part of the procedure with its flexibility and mobility. All techniques are *rhythmical*, i.e. differentiated according to clearly established qualities that are *polar opposites*. It is done by increasing and decreasing, i.e. increasing intensity of contact and relaxation, by going in deeply and coming away and expanding. The *moment of turning* from one phase to the other comes as the hands relax between increasing intensity and relaxation, and bring in the surrounding areas between relaxing and increasing intensity. The process keeps changing, with *flexible adaptation* to the given body region and in accordance with the therapeutic goal.

Warmth plays an important role. We only uncover the part of the body which is being treated at the time and work with warm hands. With every treatment we count on a reaction from the body's warmth organization.

Rest is particularly important after the procedure, even if this took no more than a minute or two.

The forms used are straight line, circle, lemniscate and spiral.

A unique technique is two-handed circles with phase-shift. Equally unique are organ treatments and the use of ointments and oils made with metals. The choice of pure natural oils and other substances is always in accordance with the presenting signs and symptoms.

Rhythmical Einreibungen mainly involve sliding movements in conjunction with

1   lightness of touch
2   rhythm
3   attention paid to warmth
4   rest after the procedure.

This essentially is what Rhythmical Massage Therapy and Rhythmical Einreibungen have in common and what brings them together.

The differences are that massage involves a *wide range* of techniques and specific treatment concepts. With Rhythmical Einreibungen, a *single* technique – effleurage or sliding – serves this field of hygienic and therapeutic nursing procedures. Apart from this, the difference also lies in the people who use either method.

A masseur using Rhythmical Massage Therapy will have had his basic training in classic massage or physiotherapy. Rhythmical Massage will be the main part of his work. Rhythmical Einreibungen are done by people belonging to a number of different professions (nurses in all specialist fields, social therapists and curative teachers) and are merely part of their professional work. Lay people may also use them, e.g. someone caring for a family member. All of the latter limit themselves to the range of part treatments, whilst for the masseur these are part of a much wider repertoire.

Massage is generally prescribed by a physician and given once, twice or three times a week, or daily in exceptional cases. Rhythmical Einreibungen are sometimes prescribed and sometimes used by carers on their own initiative. They are given daily, several times a day, and in rare instances only once a week. The reasons for this will be given below.

3   Definition of Rhythmical Einreibungen

Nursing care is part of the therapeutic spectrum. Rhythmical Einreibungen are part of nursing. In this sense they are a therapeutic nursing procedure. Their rhythmical quality makes them a central, healing, helping measure, as will be clear, it is hoped, from what follows.

One way of defining the method might be: 'A substance (oil, emulsion, ointment …) is applied to the skin with sliding movements and a quality of touch that moves between the extremes. The movement of the hands takes its orientation from the laws of rhythmical processes in nature and in the human being.'

It seems simple. Wouldn't anyone be able to do it? Yes and no. Yes, the way a mother touches her child in a healing, comforting and soothing way to take away fear or pain or bring on sleep. No, because one often finds it difficult to do the same for strangers, especially if there are additional stresses such as being in a rush, having too much to do, or not being in sympathy with the person. Yes and no, for a mother is not aware that she is using *rhythm*. What she does is rhythmical because she uses her hand lightly and yet firmly and with certainty, and then lets go again. The hand is completely relaxed, with the movement coming from a free upper arm. The mother's inner attitude and her intention to comfort the child give her hand the power of expression that is needed, and this is conveyed in a way that carries conviction. She may perhaps also hum a bit of a tune and this relaxes both her and the child. The whole 'treatment' is of a piece and yet inwardly differentiated. It is not easy to do such a thing deliberately. And a mother wanting to do it on purpose would have to learn how to do it in a completely new way.

For members of the caring professions it is necessary to become fully aware of the quality of this natural process, making it objective so that

• independent of your prevailing mood or state, you will be able to use it even under stress and

• you can use the different possibilities to specific effect.

The term 'rhythmical' indicates that it is not a mechanical technique but something which takes its orientation from the laws that govern the sphere of life (see Chapter 1, 2.5). Rhythms are processes in the natural world that are not guided by human actions or thinking but by cosmic spiritual powers within and outside the human being (see Chapter 1, 3.3.3). In deliberately using rhythm with something, we add a new rhythm, one that has not existed before, to the rhythms of nature. We create culture.

It cannot be denied but that this demanding work calls for responsibility. Experience gained in education (Waldorf and curative education [Heimann 1989]), pharmaceutics (rhythmical methods in the manufacture of medicines), agriculture (biodynamic agriculture, making compost preparations) and therapies (eurythmy therapy, speech, art therapy, social art) have borne out that rhythmical processes give strength and health, maintain and build up. Scientific investigations have shown the laws on which every rhythmical process is based [Hauschka 1984, Hildebrand 1986, Hoerner 1978, Klages 1944, Schwenk 1976].

In molecular biology it has been found that every intra- and intercellular movement is not only rhythmical but follows a lemniscate. On the one hand this is a form of movement in the sphere of life and on the other it is an image reflecting a process where balance is found between two polar opposites whilst also maintaining them.

Human health depends on rhythmical processes continually creating balance between the polar opposites active in the body or keeping them apart where necessary (see Chapter 1, 3).

This health-giving activity needs permanent support. Rhythm always contributes to it, but anything that goes against it will cause sickness or injured feelings. As a rule, the healthy organism has a marked ability to compensate.

However, the effects of anything that goes against health tend to show themselves not immediately but only after a long time. When the individual limit has been passed and sickness develops, rhythmical measures will prove beneficial and healing. Such measures include

- a good balance between sleeping and waking
- reasonable alternation between rest and movement
- alternating between concentration and relaxation
- regular, freshly cooked meals
- walking or swimming
- activities in the arts and/or art therapy as breathing processes with colour, form and sound
- Rhythmical Massage Therapy and baths
- any physical touch that has rhythm, e.g. Rhythmical Einreibungen

The necessary activity thus consists in

- either consciously entering into a *given* rhythmical process in *nature*
- or creating a *new* rhythmical process and therefore *culture*.

Rhythmical Einreibungen are a cultural activity learned from natural processes and added on to them. Their significance lies in touching the human body with the powers of general health and healing in mind, so avoiding injurious elements and helping to balance them out.

In modern life, knowledge of the importance of rhythm is either getting lost or proving difficult to apply (working nights or on Sundays – disruption of night-and-day rhythm, fast food – lack of rhythm and culture in the way we eat, disposable items – no more regular care and cultivation of things because of over-abundance …). Many people in Western society therefore suffer from rhythm disorders in varying degrees. By providing care that is in harmony with human nature we endeavour to counter this negative tendency, offering health-giving, rhythmical qualities and processes to an organism that is subject to much irritation.

The view of the human being on which these ideas are based may be found in Rudolf Steiner's anthroposophy. 'This sees every human being as an individual who is in a lifelong learning process as he comes to terms with himself, other people and the environment. In nursing, this means supporting and accompanying healing processes and progressive development in body, soul and spirit through the encounter with the patient.' (Guiding principle for trainers in Rhythmical Einreibungen).

Carers need an instrument and a technique for this mediating activity. *One* possible way is this: The hands are the instrument and Rhythmical Einreibungen are the technique which comes 'to hand'. Touch handled in a conscious way addresses the patient's powers of self-healing and strengthens them thanks to the rhythmical element.

4   Quality criteria

4.1   General

'Quality' here refers in the widest sense to everything which contributes to giving rhythmical expression to the Einreibungen. Chapter 1 provided the basic insights needed for using touch in a rhythmical way. We will now consider the way in which these are brought to bear in practice.

The order given to this section relates to the fourfold nature of the human organism (see Chapter 1, 2).

1 Working with the force of *gravity* or the phenomenon of *weight*.
   – Where does gravity have its justification in Rhythmical Einreibungen?
   – How do we overcome it, so that it does not interfere with the process?
2 Next comes the question as to how we generate *a living quality*, flow and flexible adaptation in our touch which will make lightness possible, as in and through the element of water.
3 These aspects must be taken into account if we are to create the dynamics belonging to the airy element, using them in a suitably differentiated way to be in accord with the nature of rhythm.
4 The fourth aspect is inseparably bound up with the other three; it is the attention paid to warmth at the level of body, soul and spirit. Specifically this means
   – a warm, awake, ordering and thoughtful way of working, taking account of the laws that pertain as well as the situation of the individual patient
   – creating a situation where one is not disturbed
   – evaluating the treatment to ensure flow of information and
   – always observing developments and keeping our work under critical review.

Added to this are aspects of the intensity of touch, the form, direction and duration of an Einreibung, and the choice of substance used. All aspects demand that we are awake, using our powers of thought and insight as we do the work.

The system given in Table 2.1 was produced in a workshop. Relationships are shown between

• the particular body of the human being
• the element which forms its basis
• some qualities of this element in the natural world and
• how this is taken into account with Rhythmical Einreibungen.

Living things cannot be made to fit into established systems. Thus 'form' might be put in the first row if seen as something that has evolved. Here the view taken is that every form has arisen from the fluid principle. 'Direction' might also come in row 4 if one considers that there are always two possibilities with direction and the decision based on particular aspects is made by the I. Here it is the aspect of direction in something which is flowing. Boundaries are generally zones of transition in the sphere of life, and this is indicated in the 'Transition' rows.

The table or collection of themes may provide guiding principles for the use of Rhythmical Einreibungen in practice, as follows.

With Rhythmical Einreibungen, the aim is always to overcome gravity (in positioning the patient and the posture taken by the carer), so that it will never come into play as such. Gravity only comes in with touch to create lightness for the patient or to make up for a lack of bodily awareness.
Knowing the essential nature of water helps us to understand the living nature of the body which is to be treated. The carer can become an instrument that will work effectively in harmony with the functions of the organism.
If these conditions are met and the carer gives undivided attention and takes a warm interest, it will be possible to use a breathing and differentiated touch that leaves the other person free.

Table 2.1	The bodies in nature		
Body	Element	Quality in nature	Quality for the treatment
1 physical body	solid, physical	*gravity*, coldness, rest, visible, measurable and weighable	touch as such, positioning the patient, position of carer, size of area to be treated
Transition		*overcoming gravity*	gesture, flexible posture
2 life sphere (ether body)	water	*levity*, lift, suction, fluidity, flexible adaptation, drop formation, flow	flow-determined form of muscle, joints and organs, guideline, form, direction, ongoing awareness, flowing movement of hand, counter movements
Transition		*balance*	empathy
3 soul quality (astral body)	air	*dynamism*, high and low pressure, expansion and contraction	contraction and expansion, line and circle, increasing and decreasing contact, increasing and decreasing intensity, alternation of pronation and supination, increasing intensity and relaxation, nearness and distance
4 I or self	warmth	*warmth*, absolute penetration, solution, widening out, movement	warmth in hands, substance and surroundings, undivided attention, interest, empathy, concentration, initiating turning moments, organization, overview, intention; evaluation

4.2 Taking gravity into account

With Rhythmical Einreibungen, we work with gravity as follows. It is left to be where it is in its rightful place, or used as required, but avoided where it proves disruptive or is out of place.

4.2.1 Positioning the patient

Aim

The aim is to have the patient lying or sitting in a secure, comfortable and relaxed position where he or she does not feel the need to actively participate.

The carer has free access to the area being treated and the intensity of touch is not determined by access to space.

Application

Depending on the given situation,

- let the head / upper part of body be slightly elevated (lying on the back)
- make up for lordosis (lying face down or on the back)

- relieve the lumbar spine by slightly elevating the sacrum
- make up for excessively out- or in-turned legs by supporting hip and knee joints
- relax abdominal muscles using a knee roll
- lying face down,
  - dorsum of foot on soft support
  - depending on configuration of spine and upper body, cushion abdomen and pelvis
  - place the head in a half-lateral position to relax muscles at back of neck
- and with the patient lying on the side, place a small cushion behind the back to give support and security
- clothing should not be tight
- make sheets or blankets and covers fit snugly like a second skin
- let the soles of the feet be supported vertically, avoiding all pressure on tops of toes, however.

Add to this the specific supports, spaces for access and positions required for part Rhythmical Einreibungen (Chapter 3).

It is a matter of using positioning aids effectively rather than in numbers. Different rules apply with body care for example at the wash basin or in other situations when patients are out of bed. These are above all

- to keep the body warm
- to have the arms supported in front of the upper body.

4.2.2   Carer's posture when standing and in motion

Aim

If the hands are to be able to follow the laws of rhythm, they need active support from the whole body. The close connection which exists means that the body takes part in everything which the hands do. In fact, the whole body is involved in practically every movement. Below, we will consider how the body can support the work of the hands.

The posture has an *inner* and an *outer* aspect. The *inner* aspect is that touch always has something to do with the essence of meeting and a caring attitude. The individual whom we touch is therefore included in the activity. He opens up to the carer, listening with all his senses. This is made visible in a *gesture* of the carer – to turn invitingly towards the individual human being. Grossmann-Schnyder also calls this 'intentional touch' [Grossmann-Schnyder 1996].

The inner aspect also means that movement – quite generally – includes the surroundings. Visible movement is always only a small part of an extensive invisible movement. In the same way, people about to meet are moving towards one another long before they are visible to one another. The same holds true for their parting. The relationship makes us inwardly follow the road taken by the other even though we no longer see him. Because of this, the carer does not assume the kind of position taken to protect the back when dealing with a load. In that case, an object is moved from one place to another. With Rhythmical Einreibungen, however, a movement which is already there is taken up and then allowed to expand into the distance.

The *outer* aspect is that one stands in readiness, so that a change may be made at any moment. It is a kind of 'marking time', loose in every joint, attentive to the patient, freely mobile, in 'variable equilibrium' between front and back as well as left and right.

Application in practice

- Stand with one foot forward, but not astraddle, with the back foot closest to the bed. This makes it possible to bend forward without twisting the spine.
- The feet provide information on the distribution of weight, which should be in balance between the two legs.
- The smallness of the step (about shoulder-width) makes it possible to have all joints flexible and change position forward or back at any time, without awareness of this being transferred to the patient. A change of position, if required, comes at around the second turning moment when the hands are least engaged and moving the body does not affect the carer's touch.
- Be free-standing, not leaning on anything, as this would cause imbalance.
- Mentally allow the weight to go down into your feet and also let it go inwardly. This will 'free' your shoulder girdle and hands.
- The natural lordosis in the lumbar spine proves an obstacle here. Make your back round therefore in this place, that is, convex (kyphosis).
- In eurythmy, this region of the spine is a 'character site' for the M sound. In gymnastics we speak of 'keeping the back straight'. The same gesture is practised in antenatal classes. The whole form, from forehead/occiput to soles of the feet, is rounded out. To avoid tension in the arms, include the cervical spine in the rounding process [Verband anthroposophischer Pflegeberufe (German Anthroposophical Nurses' Association) 1993].
- Your shoulder girdle feels free and open, so that movements – mentally seen as coming from outside – can be guided by a free upper arm.

- Both legs are weight-bearing and free to move, i.e. they take the weight, bear, are well 'earthed', and are also always ready to change, the joints being flexible.
- Movement is not impeded by furniture or any objects on the floor.
- A dangling necklace, scarf, long hair, wide sleeves, etc. will also get in the way and must therefore be avoided, so that there will be no need to compensate by moving the head or arms.

What other ways are there of counteracting the effects of gravity? This has subtle effects even as the contact made with your hand or hands increases. The aim is to prevent this intensification from feeling heavy to the patient. The best way of being free to determine the intensity of touch is to let your body 'distance itself' from the arm movement and include a *counter movement*, however subtle, perhaps even just in thought. Otherwise the weight and strength of your body and temperament will influence your hands as they work. In creating this distance, let your wrists be regions through which movement impulses flow. They are not deflected nor given a slant. The feeling is as if the hands extended to the elbow joints. Distancing yourself like this also protects you from exhausting your energies, however much you are there for the patient.

All in all, move your body as little as possible and as much as is needed. A mobile equilibrium results if gravity is overcome. A relaxed posture is the precondition if you want to be there for the person you are treating, with empathy in both an inner and an outer way.

4.2.3   The free hand

When an Einreibung is done with one hand, the other hand appears to be inactive. It does, however, enter wholly into the evolving process. It is always in contact with the patient's body. This makes the care you give to the patient complete. If the hand were somewhere else, e.g. hanging down or used to support yourself, your posture would not be free and in equilibrium. Place the free hand so that it does

not impede the working hand or limit the way you stand and move — especially in the region of shoulder and chest. The hand quietly maintains warm contact which continues even when the working hand lets go and moves through the air as a form is about to be repeated.

In a very few situations the free hand lifts or supports a body part (when treating an arm or foot) or provides stability (treating the back of a sitting person). It is then just as relaxed as when used in treatment. It does not take hold, nor does it tense. Use mainly the palm of the hand, making the fingers part of its surface, merely signalling gentle presence.

When you change hands, let them interplay in such a way that separation and new approach are fluid and simultaneous (treating the forearm, elbow and upper arm).

The free hand must be relaxed so that it may 'listen carefully' to the working hand.

4.3   Attention to lightness of touch

The suggestion made in section 4.1.1 is to work with physical gravity in such a way that it is either eliminated or — in the truest sense of the word — carries no weight. This was with reference to *preparing* for the next step, letting powers of lightness, buoyancy, develop.

Looking at the human body we would have to say that it is really more light than heavy. If gravity were to dominate, all physical matter would drop out of the context of life, lymphatic and venous circulation would cease to function and collapse immediately, joints would stiffen and all movement be impossible. Human beings would in fact be unable to exist.

The predominance of levity is an absolute precondition for all life forms. This is evident from the facts that

- 75% of the human body is water, the physical vehicle for the etheric powers of life,
- during embryonic development, all tissues are still fluid, primarily on the move without any visible impetus from outside, and
- the configuration of many organs, especially the muscles in our extremities, can be seen to

have evolved out of a fluid state. The streamlined form, the fact that all muscle fibres run between origin and insertion, and the extension and contraction of muscle fibres remind us of this. The last of these does, however, also indicate the influence of a dynamic principle relating to both form and function. Transitions are always fluid in life.

4.3.1   Guideline/orientation line

In the course of muscles in the extremities we distinguish a middle or main stream – as in a river bed – and a marginal stream. In Rhythmical Massage as indicated by Dr Ita Wegman, the midstream direction is called the 'guideline'.
   '... guidelines, which in the extremities generally follow the course of muscles, and even more the sculpted form of the human body ...'
   '... guidelines generally follow the flowing lines of the muscles ...'. [Hauschka 1984]
   These invisible guidelines can be seen, for instance, in the configuration of the lower leg or arm. They run between insertion and origin, not exactly in the centre but according to the flowing or sculpted form of the muscle. The hand follows the guideline's course, generally with its mid-line (see Fig. 10). This gives you living experience of your touch being 'right'.
   Rhythmical Einreibungen are not, of course, limited to the extremities with regard to guidelines. The remaining pathways are called 'orientation lines'.
   Examples are

- the course of a muscle in the trunk; not being in an extremity it also indicates the way and direction, e.g. the M. erector spinae (longissimus)
- the route around a joint where no muscle takes this circular route, e.g. in the heel or part of the knee joint
- routes on the body where either an organ or other structures indicate the way, e.g. on the abdomen or thorax
- the route the hand takes on leaving the guideline to complete a circle or spiral that has been started, as with treatments for the forearm, lower leg and thigh.

Straight line and *curve* are an archetypal polarity which we find in all spheres of life (see Chapter 1, 5.2.2). The same characteristics may be seen in the contrast between midstream and marginal flow in a river, the first being fast, straight ahead and purposeful, the other slow, rounded, and going in every direction. We can say the same about the contrast between guidelines and orientation lines of muscles in the extremities. The contrast then also shows itself in the quality of touch – increasing intensity and increasing contact over the guideline, and relaxation, reducing contact on leaving the guideline.

We get the following pairs of terms

straight	→ curved
main or midstream	→ marginal flow
guideline	→ orientation line
increasing intensity	→ relaxation
Exception: greater intensity may also be on an orientation line	→ Exception: relaxation may also be on a guideline.

4.3.2   The relaxed hand

The dominance of the fluid element in the human body is taken into account in the way we touch. Water is laminar as it flows and glides, shearing with and against itself in the finest of layers. This property enables it to adapt elastically to anything, with no will of its own – to any impression or influence due to wind, obstacles or gradients.
   Observing flowing water and studying flow helps us to develop a flowing touch with our hands.
   'Water does not want anything for itself; it gives itself to everything and never asks about the form which it is to assume. It 'relinquishes all claims' and, having served as a mediator, steps back again in readiness for new activity and mediation.' [Schwenk 1976]

Nothing softer and more yielding in the world than water.
Nothing more powerful to bring down even the strong and firm –
Invincible, for always adapting.

True, all the world knows that
the weak overcomes the strong,
and softness frozen rigidity,
yet none will act accordingly.

Lao Tse [Sandkuehler 2000]

With the Rhythmical Einreibungen, we do nevertheless endeavour to act accordingly. The question is, how?

There are two extremes to sliding movements.

1 Either the hand is heavy and clinging, pushing tissue along (oppressive),
2 or it is so light that the individual who is touched feels that it is not actually there, but floats across (tickling, cool, fleeting).

In either case the hand is not relaxed but tensed, in one case applying pressure, in the other being too cautious. This must be avoided.

How, then, is it possible to have lightness combined with presence. How do we manage not to oppress when effecting the necessary increase in intensity and not to abandon as we let go?

This quality arises quite naturally, though unconsciously, when a loving hand is used to give comfort. In the absence of such a spontaneous human relationship the hand must be used consciously if this quality is to develop in any given situation.

It helps if we understand functional threefold nature. Due to the polarity between neurosensory processes and those in metabolism and will, the presence of one always limits the other. Thus it is only possible to increase the sensitivity of the hands by holding back the sphere of metabolism and will. Too much activity in that sphere will inhibit sensory perception or reduce it to a minimum.

It also touches on a person's sphere of individual freedom if we impose our will too much [Kühlewind 2000]. This cannot be wholly avoided when we use touch, but knowing about it we may endeavour to be as gentle and careful, of good will (in the truest sense of the word) and restrained as possible.

What do we need to do?

1 Assume the posture which has been described.
2 Avoid using the weight of your hand, so that the patient's body will not be burdened.
3 Move the hand without using the voluntary muscles. This alone enables you to hold back the will and so enhance sensitivity.
4 *Intentional tension* remains, expressing interest and awareness. Lightness of touch and full attention are combined in this and the resulting touch is relaxed and yet fully present. (Intentional tension is the kind of tension one has in a watchful eye, for instance [Witzenmann 1989]. It does not arise from tensing the extraocular muscles but has its basis in our interest. This determines the specific direction and expression of the eye.)

How can this be brought to realization?

Hands change position in space because of arm movements. As their muscles do *not have to do work* to bring a movement impulse to realization, the hands can be quite relaxed, leaving this work to other parts. These are

- the upper arm, moving the hand forwards and back from the shoulder, and
- the elbow; alternating between pronation and supination makes it possible to move around and envelop the parts of the body you are treating.
- The wrist lets these impulses flow through it, moving only in flexible adaptation.
- Moved by the arm, the wrist is anteflexed or straight, which keeps the tissue of the palm more relaxed and soft.
- Movement thus does not come from the wrist but from further away, from the shoulder girdle. (Compare this with activities and movements of all kinds, e.g. cutting down trees, sawing wood, sowing, mowing, playing the violin or cello, conducting or the way a blind person feels his way.)
- A relaxed hand is able to adapt to the given forms of the body, allowing them to form it rather than reproducing them. A knee joint, for instance, shapes the hand that works on

it according to its size and configuration (see balloon exercise, Section 10.1).

4.3.3   Ongoing awareness

Being relaxed to this degree does hold the danger of the hand, which is 'asleep' as it were, growing heavy and a burden.

It is therefore necessary to 'come awake' in the hand, i.e. send perceptive *awareness* into it. Only then will the hand begin to be responsive in its touch. Considering the fact that the body is more than 75% water, we make the hand's approach like that to the surface of water, sensing

1   the subtle resistance offered to the hand
2   the suction effect as it wants to come away, and
3   the possibility of accommodating the hand snugly, without it getting heavy or falling into gravity
4   that you are supported.

The hand begins to come alive in this way, and this can be further differentiated and enhanced by focusing attention not on the whole hand at once but in subtle dosage and an ever-changing way, so that your attention will continually flow and be ongoing through the hand. It can also 'jump', of course, e.g. when changing direction or at the turning moments, but without breaking the flow of movement (for learning the technique in practice, see the exercise for ongoing awareness, 10.2).

Fundamentally, distinction is made between three kinds of ongoing awareness.

1   In conjunction with the *change in your hand's area of contact* as this increases or decreases. Starting with the point of first contact, let your attention flow to what will be the next area of contact, inwardly letting go of the one that went before. Parallel to this, your subtle intentional tension will also flow from one area of contact to the next. The rest of the hand will thus be free of intentional tension and also of any active, voluntary muscle tension. Awareness can flow through the hand in various directions,

   – from the finger pads to the base of the hand and vice versa
   – from the edge of the little finger to the thumb/index finger, and vice versa
   – *against* the direction in which the hand is moving in all phases of increasing intensity
   – *with* the direction in which the hand is moving in the relaxation and concluding phases when treating the thigh, forearm and upper arm.

2   Attention may also move on without changing the hand's contact area, i.e. with *contact remaining the same*
   – when circling one-handed on the back, with the patient sitting, so that it circles with the hand in the direction in which it is moving
   – when the area is too small for a sliding movement – on a very narrow back.

3   When increased intensity of contact is applied to tissue locally and the hand is *deliberately* not sliding but remaining in one place, attention moves with the tissue as intentional tension increases – in the phase of down strokes (on the back, abdomen or foot) with its increasing intensity.

With this kind of flowing movement quality, it is possible to adapt flexibly to any part of the body, fitting it like a second skin. The technique, always moving, flowing and changing, allows us to pay increasing attention. It is indispensable, for without it, our touch would grow heavy and tissues would be displaced. The patient would feel under pressure in that case.

4.3.4   Counter movements

We will now consider a kind of counter movement which is different from the one connected with our posture (4.1.2). It is more subtle and not outwardly visible, for it is part of our inner experience.

•   At the level of sensory perception
   As the hands touch, they perceive something of the consistency – warmth, tissue tension,

skin qualities, e.g. smooth, rough, hairy, damp, dry.

• During the treatment

The carer tries not to think of her own movement at all and to imagine that the body part in question is coming to meet the hand or hands as contact increases. When the hand or hands let go, she imagines the body part to be moving away again.

As with a musical interval, the *in-between* is gaining in significance. The person who is touched is no longer merely passive, nor is the carer the only one to be active. Both are involved, as in a meeting. It is a process of *sharing*. This brings a life into the movement of the hands which comes close to the essential nature of water and of the etheric, for very fine layers always move against one another in water [Bockemuehl/Schad 1977]. In the etheric sphere, the force always goes in the direction opposite to physical gravity.

It should be noted at this point that

• paying attention to the guideline
• working with a relaxed hand
• ongoing awareness and
• experience of the counter movements

do not yet bring rhythmical quality to expression. They are preparatory and will make it possible to have dynamic/rhythmical differentiation – just as dealing with gravity is a way of preparing for levity.

4.4   Direction

There are general and special aspects to the direction given to the Einreibungen.

In nursing, the *general* aspects are as follows.

• With regard to the development of the human body,
   – the whole human form develops from the head to the feet (caudally). This is the fundamental incarnation gesture of the human spirit.
   – the limbs of the embryo radiate inwards

as they develop, i.e. starting from the buds of hands and feet, and therefore from periphery to centre (centripetal).

• With regard to the processes involved,
   – the focus of metabolism is located towards the feet (caudal)
   – that of the neurosensory system in the head region (cranial).

• With regard to the function of organs, e.g. the course of the large intestine (clockwise).

• With regard to ether currents, the currents of life in the human body respond with a counter movement when physically addressed (v.i., Back).

Direction has to be considered for

• part Einreibungen (treating a part of the body), or
• treatment sequences.

Examples of part Einreibungen

• Treatment of the back – generally in a caudal direction
   – in accordance with human development going from head to toes
   – to show metabolism its proper caudal direction and so relieve the head
   – to address the etheric counter stream by touch going in a caudal direction
   – thus to stimulate human uprightness.

• Treatment of the chest – round movement coming from the direction of the head.
   – in accordance with the development of the human form from head to feet, and
   – to avoid burdening the neurosensory sphere.

• Treatment of an arm – centripetal
   – starting with the hand, which is in accordance with inward-radiating limb development.

• Treatment of a leg – centripetal
   – starting with the lower leg, which is in accordance with inward-radiating limb development.
   – The foot is treated at the end of the leg Einreibung.

- Treatment of a foot (at the end of a leg or whole-body Einreibung)

  Feet hold a special position compared to hands (outwardly and inwardly). By treating them last, we say the following:

  - In the foot, we are once more addressing the whole human being.
  - This sums up the whole treatment and brings it to a conclusion.
  - The feet are the opposite pole to the head, and the effect is downward.
  - An incarnating gesture arises due to the feet's natural connection with gravity and to the stimulation of warmth and awareness in the feet.

- Treatment of the abdomen. The movement is circular, following the direction of motor function in the large intestine. This is the general direction for functions in the gastrointestinal tract.

Examples of Einreibung sequences

- Leg Einreibung: lower leg – knee – thigh – foot.
- Whole-body Einreibung: the main direction is from the head to the feet, though observing the sequence given for the extremities. Observing this general point of view, we treat the back – left arm – right arm – chest – abdomen – right leg – left leg – left foot – right foot.

One exception to the general aspects concerning direction is the treatment of the *lower leg*, for this may also be done in a *downward* direction. It has already been mentioned in the section on intensity of touch that people today mostly need relief in a downward direction. It is particularly helpful to treat the calves with downward movements in cases of migraine, asthma or a tendency to develop asthma, and of a particular form of sleeplessness (unable to let go, too much caught up in the senses).

The downward effect also comes into play, however,

- when a treatment is entirely *local* and therefore not going in the direction of the head

- when the leg Einreibung *sequence is changed* to thigh – knee – lower leg – foot (the principle used in rhythmical massage)

- or when the feet only are treated.

4.5   Forms

Essentially two forms are used with the Einreibungen – a sliding movement or straight line, and the circle or round form (see Chapter 1, 5.2.2) and combinations of the two. The polarity of the two forms corresponds to the polarity of a rhythmical process. Always used in alternation they serve to bring this process to expression. If an Einreibung is given with only straight strokes or circles, these are given inner differentiation by increasing and decreasing contact or intensity of touch.

Always let the body tell you when it is time to change from one to the other, and also when the dynamic change between increasing intensity and relaxation should come in a sliding movement or circle. Table 2.2 shows the most common Einreibungen with reference to the forms used.

4.5.1   Straight line

The essence of this is that the direction is unequivocal. This gives the touch a streaming, accelerating effect in a definite direction. Along a muscle, this main stream corresponds to the guideline, and in the dynamics of the rhythmical process to the process of increasing intensity. The hand therefore follows the muscle, and in the phase of increasing intensity the guideline.

It has to be said, however, that there is *not a single exact straight line* in the whole body. Every bone, muscle or surface that may at first sight seem to be straight will on careful consideration be found to be curved (convex, concave or both). The result is that as the hands follow the curving forms of the body in flexible adaptation, all so-called straight paths assume some degree of roundness (curvature).

Table 2.2 Forms of Wegman/Hauschka Einreibungen			
	Linear form	Circular form	Circle/spiral
one-handed	• Applying substances to lower leg, forearm, upper arm, back when sitting, back when lying down • Back when sitting – intensity phase • abdominal down stroke • foot down stroke	• Elbow • Heel • Chest (2/3) • Back when sitting – relaxation phase	• Forearm • Lower leg
two-handed – same direction	• applying substance to thigh • two-handed strokes on foot • down stroke on back paravertebral in flanks	• shoulder • abdomen • knee • hands	• back, lying down • thigh
two-handed – opposite directions	• circling ankles, part 1 of relaxation	• circling ankles, increasing intensity phase part 2 of relaxation	

Your *intention* also determines the character of the movement – whether it will be particularly straight or more rounded. Depending on the location and intention, we can give more expression to the flowing quality (e.g. when doing the paravertebral down strokes) or avoid it altogether (e.g. when applying a substance to the arms). Increased perceptiveness and awareness during the treatment will soften the flow-stimulating effect.

Applying substances
Substances are applied when the form of an Einreibung is not repeated in the same location but a route is followed as on the back, forearm and upper arm, or the lower leg and thigh. These involve linear movement, avoiding any kind of streaming.

Down strokes
One-handed treatment on the back involves linear movements only in the phase of increasing intensity. It is helpful to think of getting in touch deep down in the tissues with the muscle stream which already exists (M. erector spini). This is done by emphasizing the direction, with the relaxed hand effecting negative pressure.

The same applies to 'classic' down strokes. In this case, increasing intensity is local, however, with the intensity varying with each stroke. In the relaxation phase you stay with the guideline. The extent to which tissue is taken along is different with each stroke. In the case of paravertebral strokes, you have a very marked

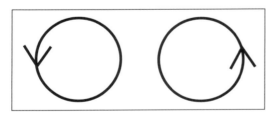

Fig. 2.1   Moving in same direction.

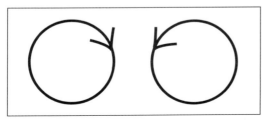

Fig. 2.2   Moving in opposite directions.

guideline which is in line with human uprightness. Depending on the patient's situation, applying increasing intensity of contact and taking along tissue may thus be very intense here (see under Intensity of touch, 4.8).

4.5.2   Circling

Circles and spirals are round, warm and soft forms following no particular but all directions (see Chapter 1, 5.2.2).

They are used
- when no specific direction is given
- as soon as the guideline is left and
- when muscles and organs present too many directions. The round form then takes in all the variety, e.g. when treating the abdomen
- when the warm quality of a round form is needed (knee, abdomen, shoulder), and
- you want to avoid any kind of streaming, and the local character of the round form is of prime importance.

4.5.3   Size of forms

This is always determined by the individual form of the patient, and there is no freedom of choice. Determining factors are
- the beginning and end of a muscle (tendon – belly – tendon)
- size of bony structures (heel, knee joint, elbow) and
- limits of the area to be treated:
  - *back*   7th vertebra, shoulder levels excluding shoulder joints, median axillary lines bilaterally including trochanter down to buttocks, beginning of gluteal fold
  - *chest*   clavicles, sternum, lower costal arches, median axillary lines bilaterally
  - *abdomen* lower costal arches, iliac crest, pubic hairline.

4.5.4   Using one hand

One hand does meet all the quality criteria for Rhythmical Einreibungen, both for quality of touch and breathing dynamics. The movement is *planar* as seen from the hand.

4.5.5   Using both hands

The hands may move in two ways:

1   *circles going in the same direction, with phase shift*. Two new qualities come into this: a spatial element that is more than the sum of two hands. The figures and descriptions given in these pages serve to illustrate this.
   - treatment of abdomen: creating a dome
   - treating shoulder/knee: cap of warmth
   - thigh: enveloping the whole of it
   - foot: enveloping like a warm sock

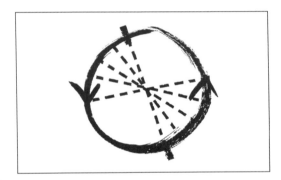

Fig. 2.3   Opposition.

Opposition of the hands creates an element of tension in the phase of increasing intensity, especially when the mid-hands are in opposition at 3 and 9 o'clock.
With the first turning moment, an inner relaxation releases a flow of warmth from the hands, and our mental image is that it goes into a spiral vortex.
Rhythmical differentiation in increasing intensity and relaxation is intensified.
   - Inward relaxation also lets the patient experience *lightness*.
   - Two hands give more warmth, and
   - double the area of contact.
2   *Circles going in the opposite direction, with phase shift*. They consist in increasing intensity – with the tissue – and relaxation where the emphasis is on direction – taking the tissue along in the first part of the relaxation phase.

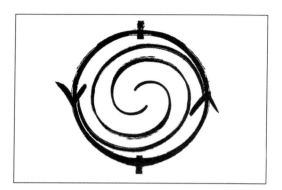

Fig. 2.4   Warmth spiral.

4.5.6   Lemniscate

The circular movements lead to a lemniscate

- always at the second turning moment – with the second loop remaining invisible, however, as the turn is made expanding into the distance and
- in the combined effect of two adjoining circles with phase shift.

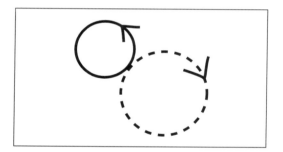

Fig. 2.5   Second turning moment.

Otherwise the lemniscate is one of the forms used in rhythmical massage, though occasionally also in Einreibung.

An accent may be set in three ways:

- downward, arterial
- upwards, venous
- locally, away from body/bone (called the cotyledon).

These are three quite specific forms of treatment that demand detailed knowledge and special skills.

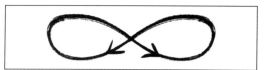

Fig. 2.6   Arterial accent.

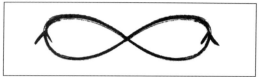

Fig. 2.7   Venous accent.

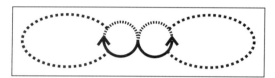

Fig. 2.8   Local accent – cotyleden.

4.6   Rhythmical differentiation

Rhythmical processes have a visible side and one that is spiritual or *invisible*, though its effects are apparent. All the rhythmical processes we are able to observe in nature, perceiving them to be the laws of nature, are not causes but effects, the *visible* part. If we therefore want to add a cultural rhythmical process to those that exist in nature, the only way is to take our orientation from the aspects that are apparent.

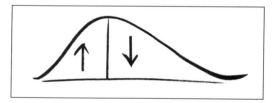

Fig. 2.9   Increasing intensity and relaxation.

This also applies to the rhythm given to touch. The phenomena of a single breath or pulse beat give a clear picture of the law governing such outer processes. It is truly phenomenal that the two phases of increasing intensity and relaxation are consistently polar opposites. The characteristic features of both are shown in Table 2.3.

The table may give the impression that mechanical alternation of polar qualities is all that is needed to have rhythm. But, as already mentioned, it is merely a supporting structure, a preparation, the WHAT, with the HOW still to be considered.

The key idea with the 'rules of the game' is: *Increase intensity without causing oppression, and relax without abandoning.*

4.6.1   Phase of increasing intensity

The phase has the following characteristics:

- Increasing intensity of contact to tissue always follows or goes in the direction of the guideline or a corresponding orientation line.
- The beginning is local and at a definite time.
- The phase of increasing intensity takes a slightly shorter time than the relaxation phase.

- The increase in contact and intensity is continuous and done *subtly:*
  by increasing contact only, e.g. when treating the chest care is needed, for you are near the heart. The hand giving the treatment is in pronation and makes contact in the direction of gravity. There is no guideline in the classic sense.
  in enhanced form:
  with a receiving gesture, e.g. treating the calves.
  The hand follows the guideline in supination, against gravity. A good muscle belly comes to meet it.
  in the most intensive way:
  by consciously applying increasing intensity of contact to tissue, e.g. with paravertebral stroke down the back.
  The extensor muscle in the back is the muscle with the most marked emphasis on direction. Being deep-seated, it does not come to meet the hand, which therefore seeks to meet it.
- Intensity is at its maximum
  – on the guideline, e.g. treating calves, forearm

Table 2.3 Characteristics of intensification and relaxation	
Increasing intensity	Relaxation
in natural processes	in natural processes
systole	diastole
inhalation	exhalation
tension	relaxation
gravity	levity
linear quality	quality of curve
with Einreibungen	with Einreibungen
increasing contact	decreasing contact
increasing intensity of touch	decreasing intensity of touch
like a crescendo in music	like a decrescendo in music
tissue under intense contact	letting tissue go
main stream/following the guideline	lateral flow/leaving guideline
straight route	round route
'receive'	'release'
supination (coming from below)	pronation
pronation (coming from above)	supination
awake in perception	perceiving as a dream
shorter route	longer route
shorter time taken	longer time taken

– when contact is greatest and closest, e.g. moment when mid-hands meet in treating a knee

– when the thickest part of the muscle's belly is reached, e.g. applying substance to the calf.

• Maximum intensity also marks the end of the phase.
• Intentional tension and receptive gesture increase the hand's tone.
• Intensity of touch (see 4.8).

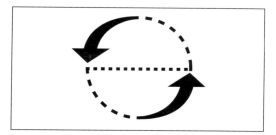

Fig. 2.10   Meeting.

'Oppression' is avoided with

• absolute relaxation, avoiding muscle tension
• a movement which in your mind comes from far away
• ongoing, wide-awake awareness in the hand
• experiencing a counter movement between the hand and the patient's body
• producing the counter movement between the hands giving the treatment and the carer's own body.

4.6.2   Relaxation phase

The characteristics of this phase are as follows:

• A definite beginning in location and time
• It always comes on leaving the guideline or corresponding orientation line
• It sometimes comes when you are still on the guideline, e.g. on down strokes.
• From the beginning, the hand is mentally set to 'relaxation'.
• Change of position in the forearm (e.g. from pronation to supination)
• The path is always determined by the size and configuration of the area to be treated.

• Duration is slightly greater than in the phase of increasing pressure.
• The end of the path is definite – either after a return to the guideline or at the end of the body part to be treated.

'Abandoning' is avoided by

1   maintaining ongoing but dreamy awareness in the hands
2   sure and full contact, with the hand warm and relaxed, and
3   gradual and not abrupt cessation of contact.

> Where we love, there is only this: to let go of one another.
> For to hold one another is something that comes easy;
> we do not have to learn it first.
> R.M. Rilke, for Paula Moderson-Becker

4.6.3   Turning moments

Turning moments come between breathing in and breathing out as well as between breathing out and breathing in. With the Einreibungen, a turn is made between the phase of increasing intensity and relaxation as well as between relaxation and the next phase of increasing intensity. These two turning moments are an indispensable part of any rhythm created. They are the core element, for without them we would not have the change between opposites. In natural rhythms, the turn comes out of the sphere of the invisible at these moments. The most suitable time is chosen, so that balance can be established in the processes. The result is healthy, harmonious alternation.

We cannot speak of rhythmical change when the turning moment comes only because one of the extremes has grown overweening, or the situation changes because of one-sided bias. That is like falling over in a faint. We fall over; this improves cerebral blood supply and we recover our senses. A balance is achieved, but in this case in a rather crude way.

With the Einreibungen, it is for the carer to know the right *time*, the right *place* and the right *way* for the turning moments (when – where – how).

Turning moments clearly show that the carer is ultimately merely creating the conditions for something which may happen for the patient at these moments. This is in accord with the nature of rhythm, one side of which is apparent, the other not. The latter only shows itself in the effect. The effect does not come to conscious awareness, however, for it is largely perceived by the lower senses (see Chapter 1, 4).

It is typical of turning moments in Rhythmical Einreibungen that in many respects they, too, are polar opposites, like the two phases. Table 2.4 shows the characteristics or polarities of turning moments.

The carer must consciously hold back her own will to create the first turning moment. This will unconsciously makes the patients more prepared to let themselves be touched. This outwardly active phase is followed by one that is more passive, though it also calls for the carer's full attention. An experience of levity also arises with the first turning moment. This is not because you are doing something, i.e. becoming active again, but because you are consciously *letting* something go (inner relaxation). We may also call it *active passivity*. This quality is most apparent with two-handed circles in phase-shift. Voluntary muscles are not involved in increasing contact, yet this relaxation can be compared to isometric relaxation. The beginning of making space and expanding comes from the carer's shoulder girdle.

The first turning moment prepares for what the patient may experience in the relaxation phase and with the second turning moment. If it is omitted or not done at the right time and in the right place, tissues are under pressure and displaced.

The second turning moment gives the patient a sense of expansion and the feeling that it is possible to relax and let go. This is the reason why the relaxation phase must be brought to its proper conclusion and the second turning moment must be given the time it needs. If this

Table 2.4 Characteristics of turning moments	
Turning moment I	Turning moment II
• place and time can be exactly determined • When: between intensification and relaxation at the end of the intensification phase • Where: *still* on the guideline or corresponding orientation line or on the thickest part of a muscle • in the process, close to the body • on leaving the guideline • time taken: a moment, scarcely noticeable in time • immediate change in intention • How: letting go in the hand, total loss of tension, corresponding to isometric relaxation • frequent leap of awareness • no interruption of outward movement • With a change from pronation to supination or vice versa: it *starts* now • effect: experience of lightness	• place and time can be exactly determined • When: between relaxation and intensification, at the end of the relaxation phase • Where: *again* on the guideline or corresponding orientation line • in the process, in your mind: in the periphery • following the return to the guideline • time taken: a moment which only seems to be longer because it comes after a long period of relaxation and going into the periphery • immediate change in intention • How: *no change of tension* in hand, at the end of relaxation the same letting-go as at the start of intensification • rare leap of awareness • movement appears to come to rest • With a change from pronation to supination or vice versa: it now takes place completely • With the 2nd turning moment as you are in the periphery, a straight route becomes a curve and a curving route a lemniscate • effect: relaxation, expansion, space

does not happen, the process gets 'short of breath', something one observes not infrequently in the patient's breathing, especially if it is someone who already has breathing problems.

Without those turning moments the whole treatment is felt to be *restless*; with them, it is felt to be *timeless*.

The effect of the two turning moments is

- that there is constant change between doing and letting be, closeness and distance
- that form and order allow the patient to experience a flowing quality
- that balance is achieved between the polar opposites of increasing intensity of contact and relaxation.

The criteria Wilhelm Hoerner [Hoerner 1978] has given for a rhythmical process are

polarity and balance
flexible adaptability
constant renewal.

Each of these aspects is valid in its own right, but they have to be brought into continuous interplay in accordance with prevailing conditions. Every stroke and every circle then becomes a new, unique creation. Every repetition is as if for the first time.

Criteria for the necessary changes or adaptations are

- the size of the area to be treated or its boundaries
- the configuration of the body region concerned – muscle, joint, organ
- the patient's needs (e.g. for warmth, protection) or condition (e.g. pain, swelling, coolness, muscle tensions).

4.7   Attention to warmth

4.7.1   Aspects

Human beings relate to warmth in a very general and at the same time also highly individual

way (see also Chapter 1, 2.8). The general aspect shows itself in that

- human body temperature is at about 37°C
- organs have specific temperatures
- core and peripheral temperature move within known ranges
- specific regions of the body give off heat
- female sexual organs lie in the abdominal cavity because they need warmth
- male sexual organs are on the outside because they need to be cool
- the kidney region needs to be protected as it gives off a lot of heat
- it is impossible to go to sleep if the feet are cold
- we have to keep a 'cool head' to think clearly

All measurable temperatures are in 'variable balance', growing more stable with advancing age.

The individual relationship to warmth shows itself most of all in the way we cope with the given laws of nature. Even infants show different reactions, e.g. one having beads of sweat on the upper lip when drinking, the other not. Many differences develop in the course of life on the basis of constitution, temperament and capacity for enthusiasm.

The connection between physical warmth and warmth in soul and spirit is evident. Children who have to sit in cold class rooms and be cold cannot possibly show the interest and involvement which is needed for learning. On the other hand, interest and involvement in something can warm up the body so much that cool surroundings are tolerated or not even noticed.

The relationship to warmth is upset in every case of illness, fluctuating beyond the usual physiological ranges. Temperatures are raised with defensive reactions and are below normal in the case of degenerative processes. Regulating body temperature conditions can therefore help recovery.

Any therapy, including Rhythmical Einreibungen, addresses warmth at the level of body, soul and spirit. It is not a matter of the carer's hands applying warmth from outside. They stimulate the body to generate its own warmth more effectively in all parts. The warmth felt through the whole body after the treatment must thus be considered to be due to the body's own activity.

It is often a question of regulating rather than stimulating warmth. Febrile conditions, for instance, may cause congestion of warmth in the upper body or trunk, with the periphery remaining cool. This happens to a lesser degree with any disruption of well-being (dysregulation of energy metabolism).

We must aim to work with all factors that influence warmth in such a way that

- there is no additional stress or disruption, and
- opportunity is given to stabilize the warmth organization.

The emphasis is therefore on everything which stimulates the body's own dynamics and initiative, rather than supplying warmth from without. The art lies in seeing when outside help is needed in the learning process which the organism is undergoing, and then providing support (e.g. a hot-water bottle), and discovering how we can help and gradually guide the process to find its own way.

Rhythmical Einreibungen are one possible means at our disposal to give the necessary impulses.

The aim is

- to maintain existing warmth and
- to support the warming effect of the treatment by the means considered below.

4.7.2 The ambient temperature

Do not let it go below 21°C, for however careful you are, much warmth is lost to the body because parts have to be uncovered during the treatment. What is more, people are more sensitive to temperature differences when horizontal (lying down). This is because more heat is given off when consciousness is reduced.

4.7.3 Towels and cloths

The materials which will be in contact with the body can be warmed beforehand using hot-water bottles or central heating radiators.

4.7.4 The substance

This is always warmed beforehand, irrespective of its nature or consistency, doing this

- with your hands for small amounts, and
- in a water bath for larger amounts. Transfer the amount which you think will be needed to a small bottle. Remove the water bath before starting treatment, as an oil-and-water mixture may otherwise be produced when taking oil from the bottle, and oils cool down faster in a water bath once this has cooled.

It is important for the substance to have the temperature of your warm hand.

4.7.5 The carer's hands

It is unprofessional to give a Rhythmical Einreibung with cold hands.

The first touch experienced by the patient is crucial for how the rest of the treatment will go. A cold touch leaves something of a cold island and does not set anything in motion in an organism weakened by sickness. This is different for a healthy organism.

The hands will usually warm up as they are working, but this is no justification for starting with cold hands, even if you apologize to the patient. The tolerance and forbearance shown by patients is often greater than can be justified. It is therefore always important to have *everything* warm.

How do you warm up hands that are cool? Here, too, treatment is preceded by diagnosis. Low blood pressure, unsuitable clothing, smoking, tension and being upset all have a negative effect on the temperature of your hands.

Ways of dealing with this are

- to correct low blood pressure (physically or with medication)
- do not smoke immediately beforehand
- wear warm clothing
- make sure elbows, feet and the back of the neck are warm
- wear wristlets before giving a treatment
- warm up a small bag of millet and place this on the back of your neck before or during the treatment
- put hands in warm water or briefly on a hot-water bottle
- practise the rhythmical process of the treatment beforehand in your mind
- with the oil in your hands, very calmly practise increasing intensity and relaxation a few times, or
- start by giving the treatment *through a towel* placed on the patient's body.

4.7.6   The patient

We cannot assume that the patient will be thoroughly warm before treatment starts. Otherwise he would not be in need of it. Cool zones in the body must not, however, be allowed to interfere with treatment. If necessary prepare and support with a footbath, for instance, or a hot-water bottle. External measures to supply warmth *during* treatment cause a problem as the patient's attention is forced to go in two directions.

For the rest after treatment, warmth needs to be supplied only if the organism is not able to generate sufficient warmth itself. It is important to continue in the quality of the hands that gave the treatment and use a warm-water rather than a hot-water bottle. The principle used in paediatrics – to offer only radiant warmth where the body is not in direct contact with the element that supplies it – is ideal.

4.7.7   The covers

Always keep the patient well covered up to the moment when the area to be treated needs to be uncovered, when you immediately offer a hand or hands that are warm. The cloths should fit snugly, taking care to see that they are secure and do not slip during the treatment. Let your movements in placing the covers be calm, not 'creating a draught'. Covering the patient after treatment, smooth the covers over the part with your hand, so that no air spaces are left that might chill.

Apart from keeping the patient warm, the covers also protect the patient's privacy and avoid oils and creams staining the bedclothes.

4.7.8   You, the carer

Make sure your hands and any substances used are warm (see under 4.11).

A warm atmosphere is created by not bringing in matters or problems from outside.

Give the patient the opportunity to feel accepted and perfectly free also to say 'no', to stop the treatment if feeling unwell, have a weep or enter into conversation (see under 5.2.2).

Create the necessary free or protected space by careful attention, providing relevant information, good organization and effective agreements made with the patient, even if the treatment takes only 3 minutes. To the best of your ability, give your undivided attention to the patient's situation, your conception of the treatment and the details required – altogether reflecting warmth in mind and spirit.

For the patient it is important that he can enter with trust into a situation of unwonted intimacy, being in no doubt but that he will be treated competently, safely, with dignity and respect.

4.7.9   Observing conditions of warmth

It will be helpful to consider this section in conjunction with sections 5.1 and 5.3.

You gain an impression of the patient's state of warmth by

- asking him about it, for much can be learned by comparing subjective and objective findings
- checking on the feet
- the perceptions you make when applying substance and as treatment proceeds

- observing the colour of the face during treatment
- observing facial expression – relaxed? ready to drop off? defensive? not feeling so good?
- observing and asking the patient after the rest period: What happened while you were resting: How do you feel now? Did the warmth continue? For how long – the rest of the day, during the night, until the next day?

Going to sleep during the rest period – even if just for a few minutes – confirms that the body has developed its own warmth.

Undesirable reactions
Sweating
- from weakness?
- too much external warmth supplied?
- rest period too long?

Chills
- from weakness?
- Were your hands cool?
- Did the treatment take too long, causing the patient to get cold; was it too strenuous?
- Was the patient adequately covered, were the covers too thin and too cool?
- Did the substance have a chilling effect?

Other observations
- Evidence of undesirable reactions also psychologically – in the facial expression, the eyes, things said, attitude?

When a patient has himself made sure his feet are warm before the next treatment and the covers are already on the radiator to warm up, this may certainly be seen to indicate initiative – providing he has the mobility and strength required for this. Or if he is able to realize himself again that parts of his body are cold and feels the need to dress more warmly – anything like this. Any change in any direction always indicates that he is putting his mind to it, and that is always desirable. It is always an activity of the I which uses warmth for its instrument.

4.8   Intensity of touch

4.8.1   Aspects

This is not an easy subject, for the subtle differences in intensity of touch *cannot be observed* when an Einreibung is demonstrated. And someone given the treatment is more likely to describe the effects of it than say something about the intensity of touch.

A description of the experience will also differ from what is actually being done, for many more factors are observed in the doing of it to ensure that the touch is flowing, adapted and harmonious.

So far I do not know of any way in which intensity of touch can be adequately expressed in figures. There is, however, one test where it is actually weighed.

Question
Does touch in which the tissue is taken along require more pressure than sliding touch?

Hypothesis
No, for the intention changes conditions in the hand to such effect that the tissue is taken along by means other than increased pressure (whatever those means may be).

Experimental setting

- a set of parcel scales (offers a large platform area)
- a towel which should not hang over the edge to any extent, so that the towel will move easily, and
- the person doing the test.

Step 1
The experimenter is asked to let his hand glide across the towel, as closely in touch with it as possible and yet so lightly that the towel does not change position or ruck up.
Result
The scales show a particular weight.

Step 2
The experimenter is asked to take the fabric along, using the lightest touch possible.

Result
The weight is 150 g less than before.

Conclusion

It is not necessary to use more pressure in order to take the tissue along. Quite the contrary – less pressure is needed.

This does not, of course, answer the question as to what really happens when the intention changes. It is, however, important to know that there is no need to increase the pressure.

Here I'd like to quote Jacques Lusseyran [Lusseyran 1963] who went blind at the age of eight. His observations make us aware of subtle sensory perception in the hands. (My italics)

'... *Movement* of the fingers was terribly important, and had to be uninterrupted because objects do not stand at a given point, fixed there, confined in one form ...

'Yet there was something still more important than movement, and that was *pressure*. If I put my hand on the table without pressing it, I knew the table was there, but knew nothing about it. To find out, my fingers had to bear down, and the amazing thing is that the pressure was answered by the table at once. Being blind I thought I should have to go out to meet things, but I found that they came to meet me instead. *I never had to go more than half way ...*

'As soon as my hands came to life they put me in a world where everything was an exchange of pressures. These pressures gathered together in shapes, and each one of the shapes had meaning....

'... moving continually, bearing down and finally detaching themselves, the last *perhaps the most significant motion of all*. Little by little, my hands discovered that objects were not rigidly bound within a mould. It was form they first came in contact with, form like a kernel. But around this kernel objects branched out in all directions.'

It is certainly helpful for us who are sighted to consider also the experiences of a blind person. We learn to touch not only physical matter but also the quality of life that dwells in it. We need

only go *half* the distance, as J. Lusseyran put it.

What is this half distance? It partly consists in the preparations which have been described above, and partly in what is still to follow. It is merely a question of being serious about the significance of these preparations, i.e. knowing that in anything we touch we have to do with the essence and that this has an influence. If J. Lusseyran discovered this from a table, how much more does it apply when we touch a human body?

We touch heaven when we use touch and feel a human body.

Novalis [Glaser 1999]

To sum up once more. You are halfway there if you act in accordance with the nature of water, the physical vehicle of life. It means that

- you are inwardly quite relaxed.
- The movement never stops.
- It is perceived even before contact is made. 'You can feel it is coming.'
- It continues afterwards. 'It goes on and on.'

Mental images that help us to create this quality are

- moving the hands as though on the surface of water
- putting them into the water without splashing
- touching the way you would if you don't want to wake a sleeping person
- mentally entering into the delicate movements in lymph vessels and blood capillaries where primary streaming and pulsation still occur
- study sound forms in eurythmy where one increases contact intensity not with something solid or water but really more with the air.
- It is also helpful to think of
  receiving and giving
  letting something flow in and out
  approaching and moving away again
- moving the hand from the upper arm and elbow and

- practising counter movements physically and in your mind.

If we only consider the physical body, a person feels addressed in his material existence. If, however, we consider the powers of life, it is these which feel themselves to be addressed.

It is a fact that like recognizes like. We therefore need two things — knowledge of the sphere of life, and readiness to work with it. Gravity will always be present in the hand which gives the treatment and in the carer's body. Yet just as dancers and actors are able to make their physical body the instrument of soul and spirit, so you, too, can learn to transform the weight of gravity.

> Stiffness must go; only the secret base line of acting in a living way shall be our rule.
> J. W. v. Goethe in his 'Rules for actors'
> [Glaser 2000]

The above also come into play in the following.

4.8.2 The direction from which the touch comes

The hand making its contact approaches the body from many different directions — from above, below, the side and anywhere in between. Coming from above it goes *with* the force of gravity, coming from below, *against* it. The patient feels that touch coming from above is something that weighs on him, even if it is just a matter of a few grams. Touch coming from below, on the other hand, is never felt to be pressure, even if a whole extremity is being raised — with relaxed hands, of course. If the aim is, for instance, to touch the lower leg simultaneously and with the same intensity from above and below, the patient will say that the upper hand is distinctly heavier.

Care must therefore be taken that the hand coming from above is always lighter when giving the treatment, so that it does not weigh heavily, and contact with the (relaxed) hand touching from below is intensified so that the patient has the impression of a continuous presence. Two examples will illustrate this:

- When applying increased intensity of contact to the calf muscle — coming in supination from below, the touch should be *relatively* intensive.
- When applying increasing intensity of contact to the arm — coming in pronation from above, the touch should be *relatively* light.

When the hands move in fluid transition coming from all sides, e.g. when treating the thigh, the intensity of touch changes all the time as the result of this phenomenon. The different forms of part Einreibungen are considered in Chapter 3.

4.8.3 Sensitivity of different body regions

Sensitivity to touch and pressure varies between different regions of the body.

Example: treating the abdomen
The region over the solar plexus and stomach is rather sensitive. Treating the abdomen does, however, take us across this area. Also, with the hand coming from above, with gravity, we need to be doubly careful. To avoid irritation, the hand 'floats' across this area.

How do we do this without losing contact?

With the heel of the hand still in contact beyond the solar plexus, the finger-part of the hand moves lightly across it. As soon as the finger pads make contact on the other side of the solar plexus, the heel of the hand lets go. Physical contact is maintained, and the hand, radiating warmth, moves across the highest part of the abdomen as in a dolphin's leap.

In conjunction with ongoing awareness this means that the part of the hand where attention lies does not touch the solar plexus. The rest of the hand, where awareness does not lie, can indeed make contact with it. It will have the necessary lightness provided that you are able to relax this part of the hand completely.

The same applies to the leaps described below.

Example: Treating the knee joint
The same technique is used when treating the knee. Instead of the solar plexus we leap across

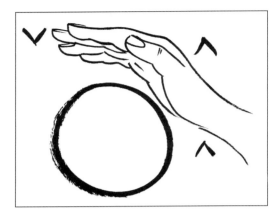

Fig. 2.11   Dolphin leap, right hand.

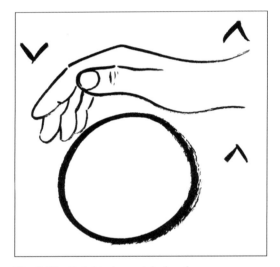

Fig. 2.12   Dolphin leap, right hand.

the tendon of the quadriceps. It is important for the hand to move at a right angle to the length of the muscle or tendon and not cause irritation.

Example: Treating the shoulder joint
Treatment of the shoulder joint, also called 'shoulder cap', is another example. Only bony and tendinous structures are in this area (including the insertion of the deltoid) and it is *the* problem area with a frozen shoulder. The hand therefore moves across very softly.

Whether contact is maintained or not depends on the relationship between the configuration and size of the area to be treated and those of your hand. If a hollow space arises, the warmth radiated from the hand will prevent cooling. If the hand maintains contact, it is particularly important that the touch is relaxed, light and warm.

Example: Treating the foot with two hands
In the foot we have the contrast between sole and dorsum. The sole takes the whole weight of the body at each step, whereas the dorsum is merely given a protective, warming cover.

Let your hand therefore meet the sole with particular intensity and awareness. On the other hand merely envelop the dorsum as with a sock or the uppers of a shoe.

4.8.4   Close to or remote from the heart

Only *one* massage technique is also used for Rhythmical Einreibungen — effleurage or sliding movement. For massage, it is used in an introductory way or as a prelude when substances are applied. The linear movement gives the technique a powerfully streaming quality which is acceptable for such a short time. The form needs to be altered for Rhythmical Einreibungen, as the streaming quality would be too much of a burden for the heart and the head.

There may be special cases when this streaming quality may be appropriate, but this does take us into the sphere of massage. With Rhythmical Einreibungen the principle is that many people today need drawing down from the head, relieving the heart, and to be 'earthed' in the feet. Changed conditions of life and work mean that too much is asked of the neurosensory system and too little of metabolism and limbs. Sliding movements are therefore done mainly in the form of circles or spirals which gives them more of a local character.

Intensity of touch is therefore relatively intensive on the feet or with strokes down the back:

- on the feet because heart and head are distant
- on the back because the phase of increasing intensity is downward flowing in effect.

Intensity of touch decreases the closer we get to the heart as an organ of the rhythmical system. It is at its most delicate *directly over the heart*, for instance when treating the chest.

It may be difficult to think of subtle gradations in a situation where lightness of touch is already paramount, but we should try and produce them. It will happen even if we just have it in mind.

4.8.5   Organ Einreibungen

Carers also treat individual organs (see part Einreibungen, Chapter 3). Here intensity of touch is used with particular care. The two most important points are

- Contact is made almost exclusively from above, i.e. *with* gravity,
- Functionally organs are even more process-orientated than are muscles, joints or bones and therefore more sensitive and receptive to every impression.

Increasing intensity and relaxation are therefore only done

- at the level of increasing and decreasing contact, and
- in awareness of the counter movements between the hand or hands giving the Einreibung and the body region under treatment.

4.8.6   Summary

The general points concerning intensity of touch are summed up in Table 2.5.

4.8.7   Exceptions and special aspects

The examples which follow relate to the increasing-intensity and relaxation phases.

Einreibung of the lower and upper arm
Intensity is very much held back in the increasing-intensity phase, for coming from above with the hand in pronation it goes with gravity.

Table 2.5   General aspects concerning intensity of touch

Intensity of touch	
more intensive	lighter
when increasing intensity	when relaxing
coming from below	coming from above
against gravity	with gravity
hand supine	hand prone
with low sensitivity	with greater sensitivity
over muscles and joints	over the organs
over/with the guideline	beyond the guideline
distant from the heart	near the heart
'earthing', incarnating	letting go, releasing

Intensity is greater in the relaxation phase, when the hand is in supination and comes up from below – against gravity.

The polarity of arms and legs comes to expression, among other things, in the hands giving the Einreibung and the intensity of touch.

Shoulder joint Einreibung, with the patient lying down
In the second half of the relaxation phase, the supine hand is coming from below and therefore makes more intense receptive contact in spite of this being the relaxation phase.

Two-handed Einreibung of the foot
To give the supine patient some experience of being on his feet, the lower hand makes quite strong and intense contact from the beginning, with the upper hand merely providing a warm protective cover.

In the relaxation phase both hands make warm, enveloping contact all the way to the tips of the toes. The experience conveyed is that of a step taken in a rolling movement that ends at the toes.

The patient feels himself to be in the foot, wholly in himself, with the resistance providing support. If the touch is not sufficiently sure and awake, the patient 'loses himself' or 'feels drawn out of himself'.

Chest Einreibung
On each side of the body contact is first made coming from above (*with* gravity). It ends on the

flanks, with the hand in lateral position (between gravity and levity), when intensity of touch is increased very mildly and gently because of the heart's proximity.

The relaxation has an accent over the median axillary line because touch is now from the side *and* because relaxation should convey a feeling of expansion. The hand therefore does not relax progressively, down to the finger pads. Instead, the finger-hand remains a surface area to the end, expanding from the mid-hand.

Abdominal Einreibung

The key impetus for intestinal activity is given above the descending colon, as this is close to the anal orifice. It makes sense, therefore, for the finger-hand to make increasing and decreasing contact *once more* after the dolphin leap in the relaxation phase. Entering consciously at the same time into the tissue will doubly intensify the dynamics (as in the evolution of pulse and breath, where systole and diastole also follow one another during exhalation).

Down strokes

The down strokes have two special aspects:

1   Intensity increases *not above* but *with* the tissues. The intentional tension spreads over the whole area of contact, causing a *suction* effect.
2   The tissue which is subject to increased intensity of touch is not relaxed at the first turning moment but *taken into the relaxation process*. This is justified for as long as the hand does not leave the guideline in the relaxation phase. This gives the down strokes a distinct relaxation, downward or concluding and limiting character. The increasing intensity of contact, taking the tissue along does, however, vary considerably with different part Einreibungen.

Every down stroke has its own specific quality, as briefly considered below.

Circles around the ankle joints

Increasing intensity, with the tissue taken along, is not local but as you move from the

Achilles tendon (calcanean tendon) to the instep. In the first part of the relaxation phase, you take the tissue with you, along the instep and towards the toes. This means that contact is quite close in spite of it being the relaxation phase. Then let your hands slide softly to the Achilles tendon to complete the circle.

Abdomen

The descending colon provides the guideline, starting at the left colic flexure in the region of the spleen. Increase intensity of touch with the hand supine and in close contact as it takes up the tissues with the mid-hand.

Taking the tissue with you in the relaxation phase calls for special skill — with the hand prone — touching from above — do not press, yet also do not lose the tissue subjected to increased intensity of touch abruptly, but respond to the softness of abdominal tissues in the right way. (Image: Place your hand on the upper part of a soap bubble so that it does not burst, and make it roll along.)

Soles of feet

Increasing intensity of touch under the transverse arch is something very familiar to the foot. The whole body weight usually rests on it when a step is taken. We will not use that degree of pressure, of course, but only as much as the soft tissues in the transverse arch and the ball of your thumb permit without making the bony structures enter into experience. The increasing intensity does already set a minimal accent towards the heel, so that there will be no impulse in the direction of the toes — in threefold terms the head region of the foot.

After the first turning moment, softly take the tissue subjected to increased intensity of touch as far as the longitudinal arch, reducing intensity as far as the base of the heel.

Paravertebral strokes down the back

Increase intensity locally with both finger-hands at the level of the 7th cervical vertebra. Take the tissue subjected to increased intensity of touch as far as the lower tip of the scapula. The essential part of the move has been done when the hand has 'lost' the tissue that was subjected to increased intensity of touch. This marks the end of it. Continue by warmly going with the existing stream, giving emphasis to the direction and bringing the size or the whole configuration of the back to living experience.

The sides
Increase intensity of touch with very soft mid-hands in the posterior axillary folds (teres minor and major). At the first turning moment, relaxation *also* applies to the hands, so that the tissue subjected to increased intensity of touch is *not* taken along. The hands go with the stream — mid-hands over the median axillary line — softly and warmly down the sides as far as the trochanters, as if recreating the shape of the body. The reason for the softness of the move is that no muscle in the area runs in the direction of the median axillary line. Instead, muscles coming from the front cross those coming from the back, so that we may speak of a *line of meeting* rather than a guideline.

Touching the body at the sides addresses conscious awareness of the body's boundaries between in front and behind and its lateral limits.

4.9 The tempo of Einreibungen

Some other aspects of the technique will be considered before we come to the patient's subjective condition.

4.9.1 Tempo in general

The tempo is guided by the respiratory frequency of an adult who is sleeping quietly — 12–15 breaths a minute. Of the two rhythmical functions, breathing has a more powerful healing function [Selg 2000].

The time taken for a circle or linear movement, which are the smallest units in the Einreibung, is thus in the region of five or six seconds. Do not check the tempo using a watch; the figures merely serve to give an idea. This tempo brings about the calm and relaxation which the organism generally needs. (The question arises if we should not find or create a

different term for 'tempo'.) It might in fact even go a bit more towards the metabolic side, i.e. be even slower, for many of the effects of the Einreibung have to do with these processes. Examples are blood flow, warming, nutrition, sedation, relaxation [Hildebrandt 1986].

The frequency should not be less, tending towards the neurosensory side, for it is never really desirable to engender nervous states.

4.9.2 Tempo and body size

How does the principle of tempo affect the different dimensions of the body?

Physical dimensions relate to three areas:

- The height of adults tends to be between 1.50 and 2.30 metres.
- Parts of the body also differ greatly from one another, e.g. abdominal or heel region.
- Dimensions also change as you move along a body part, e.g. in the calf from the slender Achilles tendon to the thick belly of the muscle.

The differences are very obvious and varied.

Distinction must also be made between two tempos:

- the tempo which in a higher sense creates a total expression, taking its orientation from the respiratory rate (see 4.9.1) and
- the tempo which allows us to come close to this higher-ranking rate in body regions of different size. It means that the tempo is generally set in such a way for an Einreibung that the length of time shows no great difference between people or also body parts of different size. Making the time ratios more the same also applies for differences within a body part.

Examples

- The smaller circles over the Achilles tendon are not done more quickly than the larger circles over the calf muscle.
- Circles over a broad back are not done more slowly than those over a narrow back.

• Irrespective of the patient's size, a whole-body Einreibung will always take about 25 minutes.

With regard to the length of linear movements and to circle size, the hands exactly follow the dimensions of the body form. When it comes to tempo, we are continually approximating. Spatial aspects are subordinate to those of time.

4.9.3 Tempo within the dynamics of increasing intensity and relaxation

The rule for the *time* relationship between increasing intensity and relaxation within the smallest rhythmical element — a linear movement or a circle — is this:

In line with the healthy relationship between inhalation and exhalation, the relaxation phase should be longer than the phase of increasing intensity, without giving a fixed time for this.

We may well assume it to be the Golden Section relationship, where the ratio of the shorter to the longer section is the same as that of the longer section to the whole. Buehler established this for the relationship between systole and diastole.

The *spatial* relationship between the route for increasing intensity and that for letting go is, however, different for every part Einreibung. The route for letting go is always longer, it is true, but it is often longer than necessary. The spatial difference therefore is not the same as the one we aim for in time. The figures given below and Table 2.6 show the time relationship between increasing intensity and relaxation.

In figures,
the ideal time relation is
   40% : 60%
compared to the spatial reality of
   50% : 50% (Achilles tendon)
and in extreme cases
   1% : 99% (e.g. with down strokes and any variations in between)

The route for letting go therefore tends to be considerably longer in terms of space, except for circles over the Achilles tendon. To arrive at a suitable time ratio we would in theory have to change only one of the two routes. Adaptation is done in two ways, however:

1 by extending the route of increasing intensity of touch in time and
2 by reducing the time for the relaxation route.

We take longer over the route of increasing intensity not only to have a sound relationship to the time taken for the relaxation route but also to avoid letting the increasing intensity be too quick, i.e. too sudden, powerful or oppressive. This is particularly the case when it is done with both hands.

To get a picture for the adaptation of tempo, consider something which every motorist knows — go slowly into a curve and accelerate when you have reached the lowest point.

How time may be stretched has already been considered (ongoing awareness, taking account of counter movements, making the circle as large as possible). To shorten or accelerate the relaxation phase certainly does not mean rushing it. The impression of being in a hurry should never arise. This is some-

Table 2.6 Relations between intensification and relaxation		
	Intensification	Relaxation
ideal where time is concerned	▬▬▬▬	▬▬▬▬▬▬
reality in space of	▬▬▬▬	▬▬▬▬
to the extreme, with all variations in between	▪	▬▬▬▬▬▬▬

thing you'll never find in physiology. The relaxation phase in particular should give opportunity to relax.

Two images can help you with this:

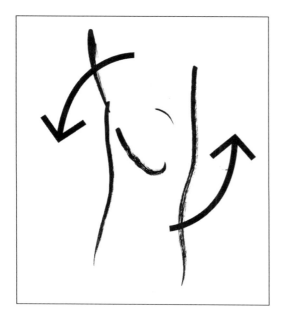

Fig. 2.13 Directions for knee joint.

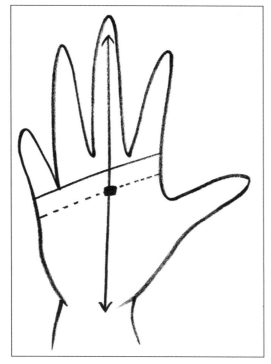

Fig. 2.14 Direction across the hand.

- think of letting something flow from your hand, letting something go, seeing something move away, or
- creating the dolphin leap; in a sense this is also a time-saving measure (see under Ongoing awareness, Chapter 2, 4.33).

It is also necessary to work at approximately the same tempo with both hands, for

- the centre of the mid-hand is not the same distance from the ends of the hand, and
- the routes to be followed at the same time by the two hands may differ in length.

An example is the phase of increasing intensity in treating the knee joint. Both hands start together – the outer one (seen from the knee) starts with the heel of the hand and therefore has a somewhat shorter route than the inner hand, which starts with the pad of the middle finger. Both hands should arrive together, the centres of the mid-hands above the inter-articular space and opposite to each other.

The outer route on the knee is slightly concave and therefore shorter, the inner route more convex and therefore a bit longer. The shortest routes on the knee and in the hand coincide and are the opposites of the longer routes on the inner aspect. It is essential to adapt here, for otherwise the situation will be that one hand follows the other.

This flexible adaptation is a distinctly musical element in the way the Einreibung is done.

4.9.4 The patient's subjective condition

With regard to the tempo of the Einreibung, the patient's subjective condition is secondary – it is rhythm which matters most.

The many rhythms found in the life of the human organism do not interfere with but actually support one another through the difference in nature. It is the relationship between them which decides the issue. The pulse to breath ratio may be the best-known and probably also most important example. Sickness is a problem of rhythm and not tempo. With the Einreibungen we therefore offer an exemplary, balanced tempo adapted to the configuration of the body in question.

In principle we make the respiratory frequency of an adult our basis, or even lower frequencies which belong to the functions of nutrition, digestion and metabolism.

Respiration and circulation are in the middle. With the balancing and harmonizing function coming from here, it is reasonable to turn to the middle and offer it strengthening support. For it lies in the nature of nursing care that we offer help to the general vital energies of the human being. Treatment based on rhythm allows us to do this in a direct way.

An exception is the asthma Einreibung given to stimulate respiration. Here the emphasis is on lengthening the exhalation phase, and treatment is entirely based on the individual respiratory problem.

Carers will also take account of presenting problems such as pain, anxieties, coldness, oedema or a tendency to get cramp. This comes to expression involuntarily in the hands – and thus also in the tempo at which they work.

4.9.5 The carer's abilities

These also play a role in the tempo used. It should always be possible for the carer to follow the process inwardly, i.e. give it undivided attention.

The consequence will be that a beginner works more slowly than someone with more practical experience. Slow starts should not be part of a nursing situation, however. They belong to separate practice done over a towel, a cushion, your own knee, in a group practice session or among family and friends.

4.10 Time taken for Einreibungen

The total time taken for a Rhythmical Einreibung covers the *actual treatment* and the *rest period* which follows. Although it is the physical body which we touch, the real 'partner' we communicate with is the life or ether body.

On the one hand the ether body is able to 'understand' directly what is said to it with

rhythmical touch. Rhythmical Einreibung therefore does not take long. If a patient expresses the wish for a longer period of treatment, we have to decide between subjective need and objective fact.

On the other hand the ether body needs time before it can respond. It is also called our 'habit body'. (It takes about four weeks for a new habit to be established.) Because of this, the Einreibung must normally be followed by a period of rest. This should always be slightly longer than the period of treatment, so that the ether body has time to accept what has been offered.

To date, the time taken is based on statements made by Dr M. Hauschka and on collective experience. The figures should provide guidance and not be taken for an established rule. They must be considered in relation to the patient's response.

- A part Einreibung should not take more than 3 minutes. The more part Einreibungen follow one another, the shorter is the time taken for individual parts. A whole-body Einreibung consists of 21 part Einreibungen. With 3 minutes each, this would mean more than one hour. It should not take more than 25 minutes, however.
- The time taken also depends on the *substance* used. The skin should have absorbed the substance by the end of treatment. The fat content of the substance is a key factor. A lotion is fat-free, for example, and therefore absorbed fairly quickly. The Einreibung concludes when the hand is no longer able to slide over the skin. The figures given in Table 2.7 therefore do not apply in this case.

4.10.1 Length of rest period

Rest is an essential part of any form of treatment. As to the length of a rest period, we again have figures based on practical experience that need to be considered in the light of the individual case.

For some people, having the rest is a learning process. There are situations where it is difficult, for instance with hyperactivity and other states of restlessness or weakness. In that case, start with a short period, perhaps just a moment of relaxation, and try to make it a little longer each time. Enforced rest makes people nervous, undoing all the good of the Einreibung. The ability to rest for a longer period may be considered to indicate improvement. With patients who are very weak and initially need a longer rest period, it may, however, be a sign of improvement if the time gets shorter.

The rest period may also be too long. The patient will show signs of restlessness or nervousness or – if he has slept too long – feel dull or numb afterwards.

It is always a case of being awake and sensitive to the issue, observing carefully and asking your patients in order to find the right length. Of course it will not always be possible and necessary to have a rest, e.g. when the Einreibung is given as part of body care in the morning or in other nursing situations.

4.10.2   A guide to length of time

The figures given in Table 2.7 provide a guide to the time required for Einreibungen with fatty substances and the rest period that follows.

4.11   Substances used with Rhythmical Einreibungen

The intention is not to add to the numerous formulae and the excellent, expert and informative descriptions given by pharmaceutical firms and many authors. For these we refer readers to the list of references given at the end of the chapter.

It would clearly be stimulating to share experiences gained in the use and actions of different substances, or to give a number of examples from clinical reports. This is planned for another occasion. Anyone who is not merely looking for formulae but would like to learn about the actions of substances is advised to gain their experience with *one* example, for this will lead to certainty and an independent approach. It is a sensible if difficult way for our present time.

Einreibungen are almost always given to apply a substance to the body. The Rhythmical Einreibungen are possible with all body-care or medically relevant substances, be it Nivea body lotion, Wild Rose or Phosphorus oil or Voltarel gel. The rhythmical touch quality and the patient are of primary importance, rather than the particular substance used. Pharmaceutical and cosmetics manufacturers with an anthroposophical orientation and many others are continually developing products that are in harmony with nature and the human being. This should not be taken to mean, however, that these are the only products to be used with the Einreibungen.

4.11.1   Types of substance

The following types of substance are used:

- ointments
- gels
- emulsions
- lotions
- oils
- essences in dilution
- milk or cream
- powder (talcum).

Table 2.7 Time taken with Wegman/Hauschka treatments		
	Einreibung	Rest period
part Einreibung	3–5 minutes	± 15 minutes
whole-body Einreibung	20–30 minutes	± 30–45 minutes
arms and legs	15–20 minutes	± 30 minutes
arms and legs only	10–12 minutes	± 20 minutes
organs	1.5–2 minutes	± 15–30 minutes

They should meet the following criteria:

- to support the skin's protective function without blocking it
- be non-irritant
- the composition and action to be such that the whole human being is addressed via the skin in its threefold function.

Vegetable oils meet these criteria. Distinction is made between fatty and volatile oils. *Fatty oils* such as almond and olive oil have skin care, soothing and warming effects. They are also used pure, especially olive oil, for its qualities are very much in harmony with the human warmth organism. *Volatile oils* stimulate the senses in many ways with their aromas. The warmth effect is more effervescent, so that they provide a certain stimulus. They are also mildly bactericidal.

4.11.2   Working with substances

The general rule concerning dosage is the less the better. Figures for some of the most common Einreibungen are given in Table 2.8 for guidance. The dosage required will, of course, vary depending on individual body size and skin quality. The size of drops also varies, as the oils vary in density.

If you get the impression as you distribute the substance that there will not be enough, take a bit more immediately rather than interrupt the Einreibung later. Colleagues with more experience will manage with less of the substance, for ongoing awareness helps the hands to slide more easily. For the less experienced the oil helps the hands to slide.

No excess oil should be left on the skin after an Einreibung. Oil has warmth nature, but would nevertheless have a cooling effect, especially if the treated skin area was cool beforehand. Skin will as a rule absorb an adequate dose in the given time.

It is different with lotions. The watery consistency means that the dosage needs to be higher. Evaporation causes cooling, and care must be taken to see that the substance has been absorbed. As soon as this is the case, the Einreibung comes to an end, as the hands cannot slide on dry skin. The time required may therefore differ from that given in Table 2.7. The same applies to milk, cream and diluted essences.

Concerning use of Einreibungen in *intensive care situations*, it should be noted that they can be given several times a day, up to 2-hourly. To prevent pressure ulcers, a brief Einreibung may be given every time the patient's position is changed to allow tissues to recover. Three drops of an oil or an equally small amount of ointment will be sufficient to give the necessary stimulus, relief and care.

Table 2.8 Dosage for substances		
Body part	No. of drops	Millilitres
half of back	15–20	= 0.5–1.0
whole back	20–30	= 1.0–1.5
knee/thigh	12–15	= 0.5–0.75
calf	10	= 0.5
foot	4–6	= 0.25
hand/forearm	10–15	= 0.5–0.75
elbow/upper arm	10–15	= 0.5–0.75
shoulder	5–10	= 0.25–0.5
chest	10–15	= 0.5–0.75
abdomen	15–20	= 0.75–1.0
whole-body Einreibung		= 15–20

Warming a substance

Metal-based ointments in a tube can be placed upright in a water bath. This will not affect the substance. To warm an ointment, you can also put the required amount on the back of your hand during preparation. Repeated warming of oils is best avoided, as it causes loss of quality. Transfer the required amount to a small bottle. Water from the hot tap will always be sufficient to warm it. Never put the bottle in a flame or on a hotplate or stove.

Rubber gloves

With some substances or in specific situations the use of rubber gloves cannot be avoided — either because the substance is too aggressive, or for hygienic reasons. Rhythmic quality can be created and conveyed even when wearing gloves. Indeed, it will help to overcome the separating and alienating effect of gloves. With or without gloves – you are always touching a person. And that is the essential basis for the rhythmical quality of your touch.

5   The whole process

This particular section focuses very much on doing the Einreibungen and should be seen as complementary to what has been said so far. Essentially the rules are the same as for any nursing procedure, e.g. a bed bath. The process is nevertheless described, for the sake of completeness. Some aspects have already been considered in detail.

Preparation
- organization/appointments
- the patient
- materials
- the room/environment
- the carer

Execution
- positioning the patient
- warmth
- protecting private areas
- quantities
- application of substances
- rhythmical Einreibung
- rest
- conversation during Einreibungen
- observation

Clearing up and evaluation
- materials
- patient
- carer
- records.

5.1   Preparation

5.1.1   Organization/appointments

- Chose a time not too soon after a meal, and one where there will be enough time available for adequate rest afterwards.
- The patient is informed of the time and length of the Einreibung so that he may plan his day accordingly and be there.
- Other patients in the room are also informed

and know that no other activities should take place in the room during that time – except for those that are essential, of course. They may remain in the room, but may also go somewhere else if there is nothing to contraindicate this.
- The patient's schedule is organized in such a way that there is no overlap with other treatments or diagnostic procedures.
- Inform your colleagues that you will not have your bleeper on during this time, as you will not be able to respond.
- A sign on the door says how long the Einreibung and rest period will be. Medical rounds, medicines, snacks, cleaning, the making of appointments, distribution of mail, visitors, etc. must wait.

Appointments are always made taking account of other patients.

5.1.2   Information given to the patient

Apart from agreeing on a time, the patient is provided with information on the Einreibung and given the opportunity to ask about anything that is not clear.
He will know that

- he needs to take care not to get chilled beforehand
- he must go to the toilet beforehand
- rest is an important part of the Einreibung. Nothing else should occupy his mind during it, not even music or a book.
- it is desirable to drop off to sleep for a short time. The carer will keep an eye on the time and return at the agreed time.
- the time given for the rest period is merely a guide and he need not force himself to observe it to the minute.
- no one will disturb him during this time. There will be a sign at the door and the telephone will be switched off.
- the carer will not enter into conversation

during the Einreibung as it takes all her concentration.

- he is nevertheless invited to speak freely about his subjective condition, for this has precedence. The Einreibung can be interrupted or stopped at any time – no problem.
- after the Einreibung he can assume the position he finds most comfortable.
- the carer will check during the first rest period if he is getting warm and feeling comfortable.
- he should not wash or shower afterwards – especially not after a major or whole-body Einreibung. The strength and warmth that have developed would be lost with the water.
- he needs to take care of his warmth organism, keeping body warmth at a steady level by wearing suitable clothing.
- he can practise observing his warmth reactions. This will contribute a great deal to assessing his recovery.

5.1.3   Materials

- The choice of materials depends on the size of the area to be treated and the sum of consecutive part Einreibungen.
- They serve to retain warmth and protect both private parts and the bed.
- Cotton flannel is preferable as it is warmer to the touch and can be boiled. Hand, shower or bath towels may be used in addition.
- They are warmed beforehand with hot-water bottles or over a radiator.
- Materials used to position the patient will as a rule be a knee roll and an additional small cushion the size of a neck roll that can be used in different ways during the Einreibung – to add to the knee roll (there is no such thing as one knee roll that fits everyone), to correct extrarotation of a leg; support the elbow for a shoulder Einreibung, and the foot for an Einreibung of the thigh.
- Place the small bottle containing the substance – perhaps warmed already – in a beaker lined with absorbent paper so that it can be put back quietly. The beaker avoids oil stains.

5.1.4   The room/environment

- The room has just been aired, and the room temperature is not less than 21°C.
- Keep the window closed to avoid draughts and external noise.
- Incoming light should not blind. Use the curtains to regulate it.
- Set up a screen if necessary if there is another patient in the room, above all to ensure privacy.
- The part of the body to be treated must be freely accessible.
- Freedom of movement beside the bed is essential. No furniture or objects to impede you.
- Switch off the telephone, radio and television.
- Have a glass with something to drink handy (urge to cough, thirst).
- Have tissues to hand (nose, tears, excess oil).

5.15   You, the carer

- Gather the necessary information on the patient, especially with regard to previous Einreibungen and their effect (from the case records, a talk with the patient, and reports).
- Your external appearance should fit in with the Einreibung you will be giving:
  - warm, clean hands, with the nails cut short.
  - All jewellery removed from hands and forearms, since accidental contact may arouse unintended awareness.
  - Hair so that it will not fall forward and obscure your field of vision.
  - No scarves or necklaces that might hang down in front.
  - Fresh breath.
  - Ensure clothes do not hold odours of scent or perfume, food or smoke.
- You develop a picture of the patient's situation and call to mind what you would wish to address now. The image of the substance to be used can be helpful in this.
- Concentration on a particular aspect of the many criteria to be taken into account can be helpful in giving the actual Einreibung (e.g.

inner or outer turning moment, ongoing awareness, counter movements). No one is able to think of everything at once.

- The awareness gained, perhaps also the question of how the Einreibung will go this time, is a great help towards being able to switch off, putting all the demands of the day aside for a while, and finding inner peace for some minutes.

5.2   Giving the Einreibung

5.2.1   Applying the substance

Only distribute the substance beforehand if a large area is to be treated. The touch used for this must also have the rhythmical quality of the whole procedure.

Application of the substance serves a number of purposes:

- to distribute it
- gain sensory perception of the area to be treated
- attune the patient to the conduct of the Einreibung, with a rhythmical quality brought to it from the very beginning.

5.2.2   Conversation during Einreibungen

You know that you must concentrate fully on the Einreibung, which leaves no room for a chat or conversation. It is a matter of diplomacy how you convey this to the patient – verbally or nonverbally, beforehand or in the process. Keeping quiet about it can cause a difficult situation to arise during the Einreibung. Telling the patient beforehand may make them feel rejected or unsure.

On the other hand a few words beforehand can ease things. Patients will sometimes only talk because they think there has to be constant talk. To talk about the issue creates a free space for which patients are often truly grateful, accepting it as a matter of course. It is a sensitive issue.

You must, of course, also know that one effect of Rhythmical Einreibungen is that people open up both physically and *psychologically*. We must develop a fine feeling for this and be able to sense if it is a situation where the patient is *at last* able to open up and tell something he has not been able to tell before. You then have to decide if it will perhaps be better to stop the Einreibung and have a talk instead, or to arrange for a talk at a later time.

This opening up may also result in the patient – generally a woman – bursting into tears. This may happen because something comes to the surface, or it may show that the patient is impressed or overcome by being given such care. We can understand this if we put ourselves in the situation of a patient, for instance, who may have been given a serious diagnosis, followed by surgery and perhaps radiotherapy and/or chemotherapy. Now comes an experience that is not in the least aggressive but quite the opposite – peaceful.

5.2.3   Observation

Before
a Rhythmical Einreibung, your observations concern the patient's subjective condition – mobility, pain, mood, mental state.

During
the Einreibung, you will perceive things mainly through your hands as regards temperature, oedema, tone, skin condition, but also skin colour and aspects of breathing. Added to this are reactions on the part of the patient during the Einreibung and anything a patient may say.

After
the Einreibung you observe conditions of warmth, changes in subjective condition, and the patient's appetite, eliminations and sleep. This applies to the rest period, to the rest of the day and the night which follows (see 2.6 and 2.7 – indications, effects).

A questionnaire filled in by the patient may round out your observations.

5.3   Clearing up and evaluation

5.3.1   Materials

- Take the substances back to their place of proper storage.
- The positioning aids are ideally stored somewhere outside the patient's room where they can be aired. Given new protective covers, they can then also be used for other patients.
- The sheets and towels are best hung up in the open air or in a well-ventilated room.
- If oil is used, it is advisable to change the sheets and towels once a week; with whole-body Einreibungen do so after every treatment. Otherwise it will be difficult to remove the oil even with gall soap*, powerful washing agents and the services of a central laundry.

5.3.2   The patient and his immediate surroundings

- Immediately after the Einreibung ask if the patient is in a comfortable position for his rest. If not, help the patient until things are satisfactory.
- A drink and the call button are to hand and the clock can be seen.
- Close the curtains further if light conditions require this.
- Depending on the weather, slightly open a transom or window.
- Consider if furniture and perhaps also the bed need to be put back into position or if this will cause too much of a disturbance.
- A bed with adjustable height must always be put back in the original position.
- The rest primarily serves to develop warmth. Ask the patient after about five minutes if the warmth reaction has started or needs to be supported from outside.
- Tell the patient when the rest period is over, helping him to get up if necessary, ask how he felt during the rest and supplement this information with your own observations.

5.3.3   You, the carer

- Having left the room, attach a temporary sticker to the sign on the door to indicate the length of rest period.
- Wash your hands outside the patient's room. This may be considered to be the conclusion of the Einreibung in an *outer* sense.
- Having cleared things away, write your notes in the patient's record. This brings the Einreibung to its conclusion in an *inner* way – though your care and further observation of the patient are still to follow.
- Reflect in a kind of review on the Einreibung and your observations. Some questions may arise:
  - Does the picture I had before I started agree with the reality?
  - Did I succeed in my aims?
  - If not, why not?
  - What would I wish to do differently the next time?

5.3.4   Records

Entries made after every Einreibung serve

- your own review
- to inform other staff when reporting, discussing nursing care, at meetings of physicians and therapists
- continuity of treatment, with earlier experiences and observations taken into account each time, and
- to make it possible to produce a final report, evaluating progress.
- Evaluation means not only that you yourself learn from personal experience but that you can also contribute this to the general evolution of nursing, e.g. for research purposes.

---

* Gall soap is a German product.

6   The effects of Rhythmical Einreibungen

Before we come to the indications, we will consider the effects of the Einreibungen to gain a clear context.

6.1   Factors that play a part

Thanks to the fine differentiation of essential human nature, *all factors* connected with the person who gives the Einreibung, the substances and materials, the environment and atmosphere and, of course, the patient's condition will have an influence. It will not be possible to mention them all in this chapter, but a few are listed below.

* Preparing the patient in both inner and outer terms
* creating a suitable environment and an atmosphere of trust
* the physical contact in itself
* the rhythmical movement given to the physical contact
* the substance (including provenance, manufacturing processes)
* the rest period
* observing the patient
* the patient's subjective condition and his needs
* the therapeutic nursing and/or medical concept
* the conference on the patient
* your training and experience
* your inner attitude
* your preparation both inwardly and outwardly.

6.2   How Rhythmical Einreibungen address the human being

Different ways of looking at the human being tell us of several ways in which he may be addressed.

* In terms of *functional threefoldness*,
  - touch acts via and directly on the neurosensory system
  - the rhythm given to the Einreibung acts directly on the rhythmical system and indirectly regulates the polar opposite organizations
  - the immediate response of the warmth organization influences metabolism.
* In terms of the *fourfold nature of the human being*, influence is brought to bear on the interplay between the lower and higher bodies.
* In terms of *anabolic and catabolic processes* (inflammation and sclerosis), the Einreibung mediates, balances and establishes harmony between the two trends. Against the background of the twelve senses, all senses are ultimately involved, but especially the lower or bodily senses (senses of life, touch, own movement and balance).

6.3   Reactions of the organism

Possible reactions of the organism include

* stimulation and regulation of warmth
* regulation of breathing
* relaxation of spasms and tension
* improved mobility
* pain relief
* regulation of general metabolism, i.e.
  - improved blood supply and nutrition for tissues and
  - better healing of wounds
* relief for the head in cases of migraine
* stimulating the digestion, also calming it
* stimulating lymph flow (in case of effusions and oedema, to promote lactation)
* regulating waking and sleeping rhythm
* relaxation and calming (in case of restlessness and anxieties, worries and oppression)
* creating trust and security (protective)

- better orientation, a clearer mind, improved concentration
- a clear sense of the body in its dimensions and/or boundaries (in case of false sensations, anorexia nervosa)
- improved well-being (where the sense of life has been impaired).

Always remember that a rhythmical procedure is never compulsive. The patient's organism must be free to respond, taking its orientation from its most urgent needs. Something may then emerge which had not come to your notice before.

A patient may, for example, be given a leg Einreibung in the morning to help him enter more fully into his body and be more awake. Instead he develops a great need for sleep. This reflects a sleep deficit which he has been able to hide until now. The Rhythmical Einreibung establishes balance where it is currently needed, not leaving anything out or letting it go unregarded. In this case, the patient must sleep before he can be more awake.

6.4   Effect on the carer

An Einreibung also affects the carer who gives it. Any endeavour to work in rhythm will also have an ordering and harmonizing effect on her. She becomes aware of this, for instance, from the fact that in spite of being very busy and involved she is able to switch off well and quickly, that any restlessness or feeling of being unwell will have gone afterwards, and she actually feels calmer and fresher.

7 Indications

Knowledge of the quality of touch and of the substances and focused observation of the patient will ideally lead to an individual result when you, your colleagues, physician and therapists meet to consider the patient and his care.

The efficacy of an Einreibung increases to the degree to which we struggle to find the solution to a clinical question, even if the result ultimately shows parallels to similar experiences or situations [Spranger 1995].

Always make sure you do not fall into deadly routine and thoughtlessness. Try to enter into every situation or encounter with wonder and joy, as though it were the first time, for

'We must go beyond phrase, convention and routine again in our time . . . – to a life where there is spirit again in every single action and our actions have not become sheer routine.' [Steiner 1967].

7.1 Use of Rhythmical Einreibungen

Einreibungen are used as part of body care, including prevention, and for special care needs.

7.1.1 Therapeutic nursing procedures

In *caring for the skin* we have to consider that it is the largest human sense organ. It is also the site for many different metabolic functions. Rhythmical functions mediate between the two. Functional threefoldness thus shows itself in the skin as an organ. Touching the skin always relates to the whole human being, and the rhythmical quality relates it specifically to the rhythmical system.

The choice of substance depends on the condition of the skin and tissues. Issues of this kind – does the skin need moisture or drying, protection, stimulation, strengthening, a healing principle – are decided on quite separately

from the procedure. The technique used in the Einreibung will support current needs, for rhythmical quality means adaptation to the condition of the skin. Many substances act on *different functions in the organism* via the skin. It is possible, therefore, to support respiration by applying bronchial balm to the skin. The substance is conveyed to the organism via the skin's *metabolism*. Volatile components evaporate and may be inhaled, and the rhythmical touch has a direct influence on increasing intensity and letting go in the breathing process.

Rhythmical touch and the substance work together in preventing pressure ulcers and thrombosis. The substance first of all benefits the skin, supporting tissue metabolism via the skin and also the venous return. For skin care and preventive treatment, the decision to give an Einreibung and the choice of substance lies *wholly* with the carer.

With the effects so many and varied, it is also possible to use Rhythmical Einreibungen beyond skin care and prevention. Nursing procedures may coincide with, or complement, medical directions. It is advisable to discuss this, so that both Einreibung and substance fit in with the physician's approach to treatment and there will be no overlaps and counter actions – e.g. due to medication.

7.1.2 Medical directions

Here the effect of the substance tends to be to the fore, e.g. with copper ointment for the feet, rosemary ointment for the lower legs, phosphorus oil for knee joints, thyme oil for the thighs, oil of caraway for the abdomen, aconite oil for the back of the neck, blackthorn oil for the arms, or *Solum uliginosum* oil for the back. This is often for the local treatment of symptoms.

Then there is the relationship of one region of the body to another, or between organs and functions, e.g.

- thigh Einreibung for digestive disorders
- foot Einreibung for difficulties in going to sleep
- arm Einreibung for eating disorders
- spleen Einreibung for weakness of the immune system.

Here, too, the effects of the Einreibung and the substance complement one another.

7.1.3   Another approach to finding the indication

This consists in starting with the effects of Rhythmical Einreibungen and relating these to the needs or subjective condition or symptomatology.
  Examples

- stimulating blood supply and nutrition in tissues
  − prevention of pressure ulcers
  − for wound healing
- generating warmth
  − for cold zones
  − if there are problems going to sleep connected with cold zones
  − symptoms due to coldness such as tension, spasms, pain, and limitation of movement due to arthritis and rheumatic conditions
- generating rhythm
  − to ease or deepen breathing
  − to tone the blood vessels
  − to regulate the rhythm of sleeping and waking
  − to regulate digestive functions
- rousing awareness
  − to clarify bodily sensations − for boundaries or for specific regions of the body
  − to support a feeling for health
  − to gain better orientation in time and space
  − to help develop trust in the surrounding world and other people
  − to strengthen self awareness.

7.2   Uses

Understanding the effects of touch with rhythmical quality, you are able to use it indepen-

dently. The examples given below are not set formulae but intended to cover the most relevant aspects in some situations and specialist fields. The whole range of uses cannot be considered in detail here. The sequence of choices takes its orientation from the biography.
  No reference is made to the vast number of specialist fields, though the method is of great value particularly in the fields of surgery and intensive care. Generally speaking, research findings are not yet available in nursing science.

7.2.1   Expectant mothers

Gravid women find the protective gesture of Rhythmical Einreibungen a real benefit. It is important for the carer to have the child growing in the womb in mind at every touch.
  Rhythmical Einreibungen are indicated for

- aching legs
- muscle tension in the back
- general problems such as exhaustion.

Substances will specifically support the effect of the Einreibung.

7.2.2   Pregnant women attending a course on Rhythmical Einreibungen

They can practise the method and observe it but at no stage of the pregnancy should they take on the role of 'object for practice or demonstration'. The organism is much more sensitive to anything at this time and more open than usual. This is even more so for the foetus; we only have to think of the fact that even moods and sensations influence development.
  Einreibungen given in a course are first steps in practising the method. They are not nursing procedures. Trying things out, making mistakes, stopping in between, repeating a sequence, feedback as treatment is in progress and discussing questions that arise − all this is part of the process. It would be too much for mother and child and thus needs to be avoided.

7.2.3   Pre-partum

A whole-body Einreibung provides a good opportunity to

- provide stimulus as labour starts, or
- also to relax, so that the woman in labour can drop off to sleep again.
- Caution is, however, indicated with premature labour.

7.2.4   During parturition

The normal birthing process may be supported, among other things, by treating the sacral region, the legs or the feet, to

- reduce pain
- deepen the breathing, and
- generally calm by one's presence.

In the birth process, mother and child are in a borderline area where the rhythmical element proves particularly effective.

7.2.5   Post-partum

Rhythmical Einreibungen can help to regulate

- involution (Einreibung of the back and abdomen)
- haemopoiesis and lactation (Einreibung of the arms)
- venous return in the legs (Einreibungen of the lower legs, legs, abdomen)
- mental stabilization (Einreibung of arms and legs).

7.2.6   Infants

Rhythmical touch quality helps healthy infants in

- recreating the protective environment before birth
- supporting bodily growth and development and organs that are still developing
- stimulating healthy development of the sensitive warmth organism

- continuing the work of the angel in the infant's body, as Rudolf Steiner put it.

Warm hands are an absolute must. All forms are round, adapted flexibly to the infant forms. The technique calls for an extreme simplification, leaving aside all specifics. The infant's foot, for instance, will only develop fully once the child begins to stand and walk. It therefore needs to be addressed differently compared to an adult's foot.

As a matter of course, every Einreibung is made an integral part of the daily routine. Humming, singing or talking to the infant may go hand in hand with the attention given to the child.

The same applies with *sick* infants, except that greater caution is indicated.

7.2.7   Children

Childhood diseases are characteristic for this time of life. As children get older, psychological problems such as restlessness, anxiety states may develop in addition to the more functional conditions and influence sleep, eating and elimination, breathing, enjoyment of life and learning as well as general well-being. Rhythmical Einreibungen still need to be simplified in the early years – round forms, brief Einreibungen, and *warm* hands.

Treating your own child helps the mother/father–child relationship. Carers are therefore happy to instruct parents in giving these Einreibungen to their child.

7.2.8   Education for special needs/social therapy

Here one of the tasks is to help the psychological and mental development of children, young people and adults by treating the body. This applies particularly to caring for the lower, bodily senses. Emphasis must also be given to caring for the warmth organism.

Both areas can be supported by a rhythmical life style and rhythmical treatments. Einreibungen and above all organ Einreibungen play a special role in this. With children, the above-mentioned aspects also apply.

7.2.9   Psychiatry

The following may be said concerning this vast field. Psychiatry seen in a wider context through anthroposophy is based on the following:

The Body as an Instrument of the Soul [W. Buehler], and 'it is always the case that the mind's ability to express itself is upset by the physical organism; it never is an actual illness of the life in spirit or soul' [Steiner in *Fundamentals of Anthroposophical Medicine*, GA 314].

The important aspect for nursing care is that the choice of Einreibung is mainly determined not by a disease label but by the presenting phenomena.

Disorders in this field essentially relate to three areas:

- warmth, there being too much or too little
- gravity and levity, with a potential bias in one direction or the other
- the middle being lost as the ability to follow the pendulum swing gets less and the order-creating balancing function cannot be brought into play.

Rhythm — offered in life style and different therapies — is the *non plus ultra*. The role of Rhythmical Einreibungen frequently is to prepare the ground for specific therapies or to make the patient more receptive to these. Much the same may be said for stimulating the warmth organism: 'A cold body cannot be treated' [Sauer 2000]. In other words, the presence of warmth is needed to reach the self or I of a person in therapy. This applies to the actions of medicines — whether homoeopathic or conventional — as well as art therapies.

Part, organ and whole-body Einreibungen, complemented by other external applications, help to stimulate the warmth organism. They also encourage healthy interaction between the different bodies (see chapter 1, 2).

7.2.10   Neurology

One aspect of this field is the dominance of gravity and coldness, with changes in the physical body also influencing soul and spirit. With paresis, you can see very clearly how conscious awareness withdraws from the area so that it ceases to exist for the individual concerned.

Rhythmical Einreibungen stimulate the physiological functions in the affected part of the body. Rhythmical touch offers the organism and the individual person something which they would otherwise do themselves in many different ways by way of movement, warming, touch and taking note. Part Einreibungen given several times a day are widely used in this field.

Whole-body Einreibungen are indicated particularly when a person suffering from paresis is to be given living experience of his wholeness.

7.2.11   Care of the elderly

With age, life progressively withdraws from the physical. This need not but may make itself felt in limitation of movement, in that many organs, especially the sense organs, function less well, and the body is no longer adequately warmed through.

Rhythmical Einreibungen can be very helpful in counteracting the heaviness which is common at this age. Problems with orientation and anxiety may cause distrust, sadness and resignation to develop, and here many occasions offer themselves when touch with rhythmical quality may be applied through clothing, without using substances. This may take the form of physical contact in the course of the day or consciously used stroking movements down the back or on the feet. These help with orientation and convey security and trust.

Care of the elderly is a vast field for the creative use of Rhythmical Einreibungen.

7.2.12   The dying

For as long as a human being still dwells in his body — which is until the last breath — he needs our help. The whole repertoire of preventive treatments is needed, and also the support that comes with the nearness of another human being. It is particularly important to deal helpfully and suitably with all discomforts, sensations gone awry, and the lack of outer and inner mobility. Worries that we might be disturbing or preventing someone from dying fade away if we work gently and with care.

Sleep, 'death's little brother', only comes when the feet are warm, i.e. the I has taken hold of the whole body. In the same way it is easier to die when warmth and hence the I have penetrated the whole body. The rhythmical quality of Rhythmical Einreibungen makes them particularly helpful in this care situation.

8   Contraindications

Rhythmical Einreibungen have no contra-indications, for the rhythmical quality of touch means that we are able to adapt flexibly to all situations in ways that are always new. It does, of course, depend on the carer's ability to produce this quality.

The following should be noted, however.

- Einreibungen are not applied to skin defects or wounds. The definition of the Rhythmical Einreibung is, after all, that it is treatment of the skin. If there is a skin defect, of if the skin is injured or destroyed, the Einreibung cannot be applied in that area.
- Einreibungen are only given with the patient's consent. To gain this and act accordingly is a key qualification and not a matter of contraindication.

Beyond this, the 'rules of the game' are not fixed. They depend somewhat more on the abilities of the carer than on the situation of the patient.

In some establishments agreements are made where the carer's abilities are taken into account. Accepting your own limitations is truly professional. Beginners therefore will not give Einreibungen to

- patients with acute conditions (e.g. myocardial infarction, stroke, rigors, status asthmaticus, colics, thrombosis, embolisms)
- patients with high temperatures (e.g. pyelonephritis, pneumonia, thrombophlebitis, infectious diseases, sepsis)
- patients with inflammatory conditions (e.g. mastitis, whitlow, herpes, acute rheumatism)
- pregnant women who are at risk.

In all the above, the rhythmic quality of touch which has been learned can of course be applied with general nursing procedures such as washing, skin care and preventive measures.

Your limits expand with practice, experience and growing confidence.

It will then be possible, for instance, to

- treat an open wound around the margins, to stimulate blood flow and tissue metabolism
- ease things for an asthmatic by treating the calves downwards.
- treat the abdomen and legs of a feverish patient with cold extremities (due to circulatory dysregulation) to induce better distribution of warmth and hence a reduction in temperature.
- give relief where a highly inflamed joint is sensitive to touch by calm, sliding strokes that do not burden.
- achieve relief for a paraplegic suffering from increased spasticity.

Your inner attitude to the presenting situation has a powerful influence, so that the classic contraindications do not apply in that case.

9   What is demanded of you, the carer

Learning to use this natural skill consciously and to touch a person in the right way does present a problem. Bringing it to conscious awareness will initially affect any existing ability. A typical example is balancing on a line painted on the floor. We wobble in spite of the fact that it is possible to move straight ahead and there is no danger of falling.

What does it mean to gain the ability in a new way?
A consciously acquired ability is not just a new skill but also a step in personal development, for it will increasingly lead to independence and creativity. A natural ability may always be lost. Something I have consciously acquired is truly part of myself (Zuckmayer – German dramatist).

Nursing care may thus become an art. Among other things, art means that a natural ability has been transformed and taken to a new level.

In this sense, efforts made to develop a rhythmical quality of touch with which we are basically familiar can contribute to nursing care as an art.

> Gradually you come to see the connection.
> But only
> because you are always actively and deliberately,
> and indeed methodically,
> working towards a point
> where something more will happen,
> broadening the mind.
> Our own activity is essential
> if we are to be given something.
>   From a conversation with J. Beuys

> Allmählich erkennt man den Zusammenhang.
> Aber nur dadurch,
> dass man immer ganz bewusst und aktiv
> auf eine methodische Art und Weise
> sich an einen Punkt heranarbeitel,
> wo etwas Weiteres geschieht
> im Sinne der Bewusstseinserweiterung.
> Die Aktivität ist die Voraussetzung,
> dass einem etwas gegeben wird.
>   From a conversation with J. Beuys

The flexibility we need to do justice to the different conditions and situations given with a Rhythmical Einreibung, using the single motif of increase intensity/turn – relax/turn, is rather like dancing, as put in words by St Augustine.

> Dance of liberation
>
> I praise the dance,
> for it frees us from the heaviness of things,
> making the singular part of the community.
> I praise the dance
> which demands all and gives all,
> health and a clear mind and cheerful soul.
> Dance is transformation of space, of time, of man
> who is forever threatening to fall apart,
> becoming all brain, will or feeling.
> Dance on the other hand demands the whole
>   person
> who in his middle is under the spell of
>   desirousness for people and things
> and the demonic nature of being abandoned in
>   our own I.
> Dance demands a free, freely moving human being
> with all his strengths in balance.
> I praise the dance.
> Learn to dance, then,
> or the angels won't know what to do with you in
>   heaven.
>   Augustine

St Augustine was addressing different aspects of the interplay between body, soul and spirit. In the last lines, he is referring to an interplay that goes beyond this, being between human beings and angels. The way I see it, we can look at this in two ways. The angels want to be able to do something with human beings when these return to heaven again, or: *the angels in heaven* would like to be able to do something with human beings whilst these are still in life, working together, as it were. For this they need human beings who are outwardly and inwardly mobile (dancing) on earth. The polar quality of this collaboration (human being – angel) may be seen as a rhythmical process.

Rudolf Steiner referred to rhythm as 'half spiritual'. The spiritual part would be the work done in heaven and thus by the angels. The other part consists in human beings on earth creating conditions that will allow the angels to take a hand.

When angels and human beings are able to do something with one another, the earth comes to be a bit more heaven, or a bit of 'heaven on earth'.

10   Exercises

10.1   Balloon exercises

Aim

Experiences to be gained with the hand completely relaxed, to

- let the hand be formed by the shape of the object
- learn to take note of counter movements
- increase awareness in the hand
- develop a living, gentle touch
- let the hand change location without being actively involved.

Method

Take an inflated balloon. Dust it and your hands with talcum powder so that movement may be as quiet as possible and slide smoothly.

1   Hold the balloon where the knot is, to keep it in place.
    The other hand faces downwards in prone position (like Adam's hand in Michelangelo's *The Creation of Adam*).
    Bring the balloon up to that hand from below until the hand fits it closely. The hand is relaxed and merely responds.
    Task: perceive the sensation for the hand when its position is being changed from outside.
2   Hold the balloon steady.
    Take the relaxed hand to the balloon by letting the upper arm/shoulder move it forward. Use the elbow to make the hand supine. The upper arm then takes the hand away from the balloon again.
    Contact with the balloon is close and enveloping, with the hand not playing an active role.
    As the hand is taken towards the balloon, imagine the balloon moving towards it.
    As the hand leaves the balloon again, imagine that the balloon is moving away.
    Aims: to leave your own movement out of

consideration and let the object you touch be part of the contact movement.

10.2   Exercise for ongoing awareness

Aim

- A relaxed state
- To bring movement and awakeness of the hand together without using its voluntary muscles

The image we have when doing the exercise: The insides of my hands are covered with numerous eyes. These can open and close independently of one another.

- Opened, the eyes correspond to waking daytime consciousness
- closed, they correspond to
  1   the sleep level of consciousness (i.e. not perceiving anything)
  2   the dream level of consciousness (i.e. knowing where they are without being able to see).

Tension is slightly raised in the opened eyes, like the extra tone in the expression and direction of an actively looking eye.

The closed eye – whether dreaming or sleeping – lacks this added tone.

Concerning the touch used with Rhythmical Einreibungen – the touch has two phases. Making contact and letting go.

Both are part of the process with increasing and decreasing contact and increasing and decreasing intensity of touch. The changes are gradual, flowing, in the most relaxed way possible. The fundamental difference between the two phases lies in the difference in tension – comparable to the difference in tension between the eye when open and awake and an eye that is closed and dreaming or sleeping.

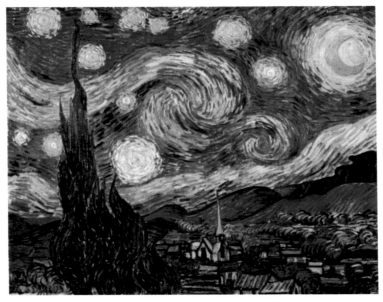

Fig. 1   Air (after Vincent van Gogh).

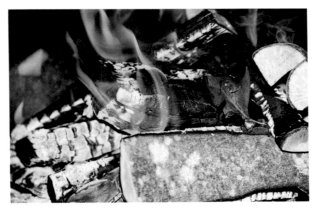

Fig. 2   Fire (photographer: Juergen George).

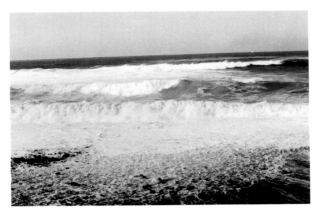

Fig. 3   Wave.

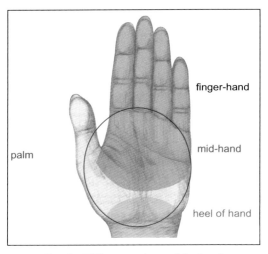

Fig. 4 Different regions of the hand

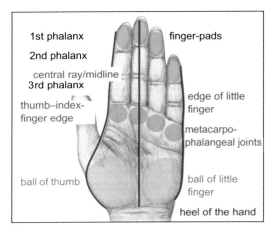

Fig. 5 Terms used for parts of the hand.

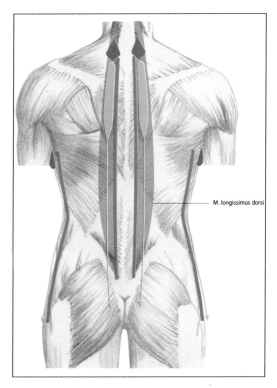

Fig. 6 Down strokes for spine and flanks.

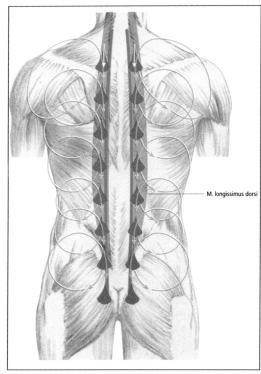

Fig. 7 One-handed back Einreibung for a male patient.

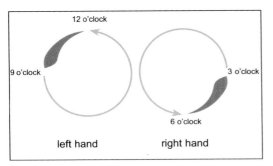

Fig. 8   Circles with phase shift.

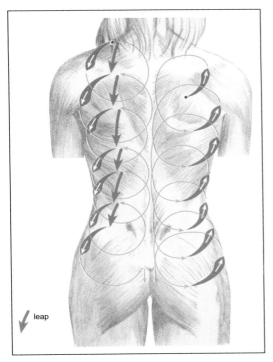

Fig. 9   Two-handed back Einreibung.

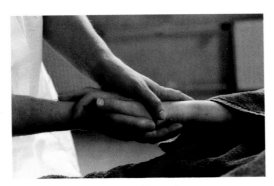

Fig. 10   Hand Einreibung.

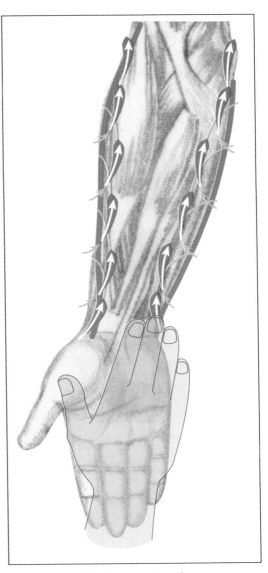

Fig. 11   Forearm Einreibung.

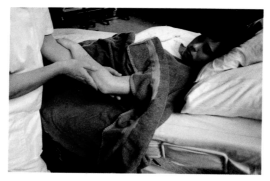

Fig. 12   Positioning for elbow Einreibung.

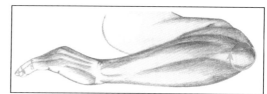

Fig. 13   Elbow Einreibung.

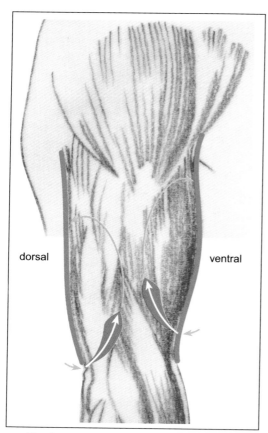

dorsal

ventral

Fig. 14   Upper arm Einreibung, inner and
outer aspect.

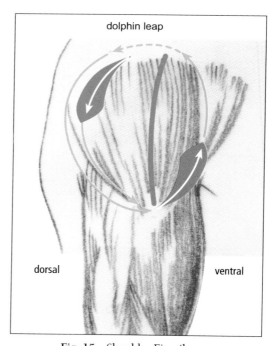

dolphin leap

dorsal

ventral

Fig. 15   Shoulder Einreibung.

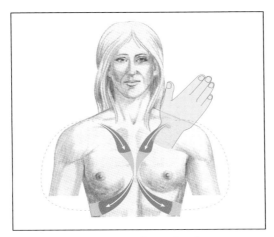

Fig. 16 Chest Einreibung, female patient.

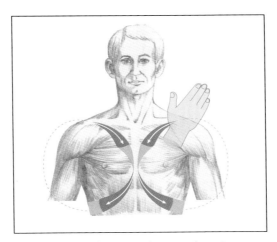

Fig. 17. Chest Einreibung, male patient.

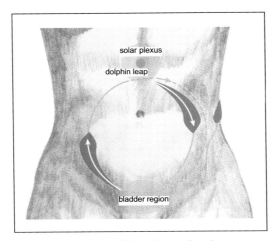

Fig. 18 Abdominal Einreibung, female patient.

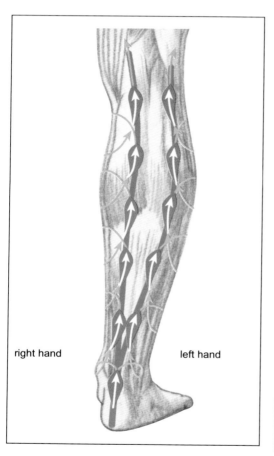

right hand   left hand

Fig. 19   Lower leg Einreibung.

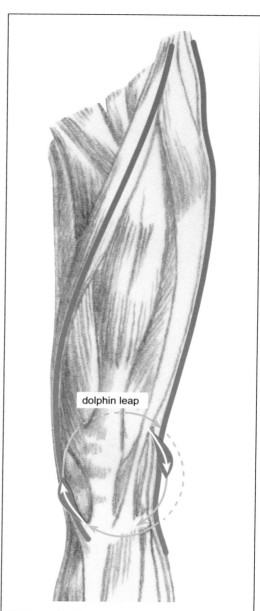

dolphin leap

Fig. 20   Knee Einreibung.

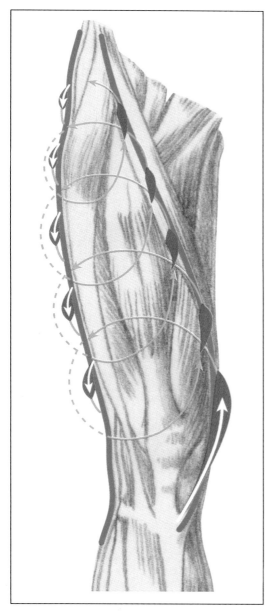

Fig. 21 Thigh Einreibung.

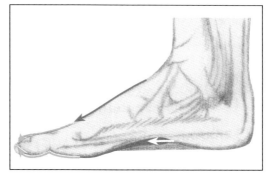

Fig. 22 Two-handed strokes.

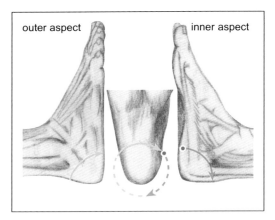

outer aspect   inner aspect

Fig. 23   Heel circles.

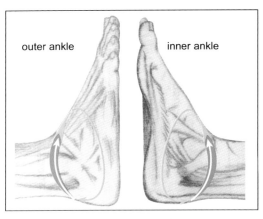

outer ankle   inner ankle

Fig. 24   Ankle circles.

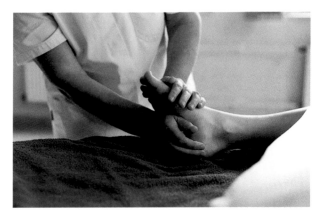

Fig. 25   Posture for stroke on sole of foot.

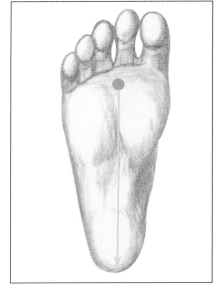

Fig. 26   Stroke on sole of foot.

Example

1   Increasing contact from terminal phalanges to heel of hand.

Contact is continually made with a new part of the hand:

1st, 2nd, 3rd phalanges, metacarpals, metacarpophalangeal joints, mid-hand, heel of hand (carpus) – to mention the major parts.

Whenever new contact is made the eyes open – equivalent to a slight increase in tension – and then immediately close again, which is the equivalent of relaxation.

In the phase of increasing intensity of contact there is constant change between opened, waking and closed, sleeping eyes.

2   Decreasing contact from heel of hand to terminal phalanges.

There is always a new place in the hand where contact ceases again – heel of hand, mid-hand, metacarpophalangeal joints, 3rd, 2nd and 1st phalanges.

Wherever new contact is made, the closed eyes come a little more awake, i.e. dreaming, only to go back to sleep again the next moment. Relaxation is complete with both, with the dreamlike waking state merely reflected in increased awareness.

In the phase of decreasing contact, or letting go, alternation occurs between closed and dreaming eyes on the one hand, and closed, sleeping eyes on the other.

1st exercise

Move your fully relaxed hand across the seam of some trousers, from the pads of the fingers to the heel of hand and then back again. The part of the hand which senses the seam changes continually. The seam arouses our awareness, as it were. The eyes in the hand open where it senses, and then close again the next moment.

It is in this sense that we speak of ongoing, flowing awareness.

2nd exercise

Let your completely relaxed hand move across a smooth fabric with no seam in it, from the pads of your fingers to the heel of the hand and back again. Send your awareness deliberately always to the area of new contact, as if looking for the seam.

3rd exercise

Like exercise 2, but changing the direction in which contact is made from the edge of the little finger towards the thumb and vice versa.

4th exercise

As contact *increases*, attention moves through the hand *against* the direction of movement.

As contact *decreases*, ongoing awareness may go both *against* and *with* the direction of movement.

Let the relaxed hand move across a fabric, making contact starting from the pads of your fingers. When contact is complete, and awareness has reached the heel of the hand, let the contact go again, starting from the heel of the hand and going in the direction of the finger pads – the direction of the hand's movement remaining the same (e.g. to apply a substance to the lower leg).

5th exercise

Increasing contact may come twice in succession – from the pads of your fingers in the direction of the heel of the hand and then again from the finger pads in the direction of the mid-hand. Having reached the heel of the hand for the first time, awareness 'leaps' from there to the finger pads (e.g. with a full circle around the knee joint). The part of the hand where the eyes are sleeping need not let go physically so long as it is relaxed in the way appropriate for the sleeping state.

Sources

Bockemuehl/Schad. *Erscheinungsformen des Aetherischen*. Stuttgart: Freies Geistesleben 1977.

Buehler, Walther. *Living with your Body. The Body as an Instrument of the Soul.*

Glaser H. Die Rhythmischen Einreibungen nach Wegman/Hauschka. Menschengemaesse Beruehrung pflegen. *Gesundheitspflege initiativ*, Esslingen 1999.

Grossmann-Schnyder M. *Beruehren*. Stuttgart: Hippokrates 1996.

Hauschka M. *Rhythmical Massage as Indicated by Ita Wegman.*

Heimann R. Der *Rhythmus und seine Bedeutung fuer die Heilpaedagogik*. Stuttgart: Urachhaus 1989.

Hildebrandt G. *Die rhythmische Organisation des Menschen und ihre Bedeutung fuer die Heilkunst*. Bad-Liebenzell: Verein fuer anthroposophisches Heilwesen 1986.

Hoerner W. *Zeit und Rhythmus. Die Ordnungsgesetze der Erde und des Menschen*. Stuttgart: Urachhaus 1978.

Klages L. *Vom Wesen des Rhythmus*. Zurich: Gropengiesser 1944.

Kuehlewind G. *Der sanfte Wille*. Stuttgart: Freies Geistesleben 2000.

Lusseyran J. *And There Was Light*. Translated from the French by Elizabeth R. Cameron. Floris Classics. Edinburgh: Floris Books 1963.

Rundbrief des Verbandes Anthroposophisch orientierter Pflegeberufe e.V., Michaeli 1993.

Sandkuehler M. *Wasser, Elixier des Lebens*. Stuttgart: Urachhaus 2000.

Sauer M. Referat vom 03. 10. 2000 am Goetheanum, Dornach/CH

Schwenk T. *Sensitive Chaos*. London: Rudolf Steiner Press 1996.

Selg P. *Vom Logos menschlicher Physis*. Dornach: Verlag am Goetheanum 2000.

Spranger C. *Krankenbeobachtung*. Stuttgart: Urachhaus 1995.

Steiner R. *Manifestations of Karma*. London: Rudolf Steiner Press 1995.

Steiner R. *The Younger Generation*. Tr. R. M. Querido. New York: Anthroposophic Press 1967.

Witzenmann H. *Sinn und Sein*. Stuttgart: Freies Geistesleben 1989.

Further reading and addresses relating to substances

Aetherische Oele. Weleda Korrespondenzblaetter fuer Aerzte Nr. 133, November 1992.

Hauschka M. *Rhythmical Massage as Indicated by Ita Wegman* (v.s.). Chapter on oil qualities. Margarethe Hauschka Schule, Gruibinger Strasse 29, D-73087 Boll/Goepp.

Hauschka R. *The Nature of Substances*.

Hauschka R. *Heilmittellehre*. Frankfurt/M.: Vittorio Klostermann 1965.

Heilpflanzen in Haut- und Massageoelen. Eckwaelden/ Bad Boll: Wala Heilmittel GmbH.

Pelikan W. *Healing Plants*. vol. 1. Tr. A. Meuss. Spring Valley: Mercury Press 1997.

Pelikan W. *Heilpflanzenkunde* Bd 1 − 3. Dornach: Philosophisch-Anthroposophischer Verlag am Goetheanum 1958.

Pelikan W. *The Secrets of Metals*. New York: Anthroposophic Press 1973.

Praeparate-Informationen fuer die Physikalische Therapie. Schwaebisch-Gmuend: Weleda AG, Heilmittelbetriebe.

Schmidt G. *Der Oelbildungsprozess*. Werner Junge, Oeldispersions-Apparatebau. Boll/Goepp.

Schramm H. *Heilmittel-Fibel zur anthroposophischen Medizin*. Schaffhausen: Novalis 1983.

WELEDA pflege FORUM; Hefte 1−4 ff, Weleda AG Heilmittelbetriebe, Postfach 1320, D-73503 Schwaebisch-Gmuend.

Weisendes und Wesentliches zu den Heilmitteln der Weleda. Weleda Schriftenreihe Heft 5, Weleda-Verlag Arlesheim/CH, Schwaebisch Gmuend 1961.

Zwiauer H. Fette und aetherische Ole in ihrer Wirkung auf die Haut. Weleda AG, Heilmittelbetriebe, D- 73527 Schwaebisch- Gmuend.

Chapter 3
Methodology for part Einreibungen

The methods given here for part Einreibungen are very detailed and more 'technical' by nature. It is important to have in mind and practise all the criteria given in Chapter 2 both when reading the text and when using Einreibungen. Readers are assumed to be familiar with these. Specific reference to Chapter 2 will only be made when there are further aspects to be considered.

Every part Einreibung can also be an element in a whole-body Einreibung. The latter is not described as it is used on highly specific medical indications. Nor is reference made to the fact that the Einreibungen do, of course, also provide skin care.

I feel it is important to emphasize that Einreibungen cannot be learned from this book. The intention is merely to offer opportunity for going more deeply into the matter after attending a training course, or to provide a reference work.

Leaving aside gender equality, and to achieve good readability, the individuals involved in the procedure are referred to as 'the patient' or 'the carer' with pronouns of either gender.

1   *Monika Layer*   Back Einreibung (Plate, Fig. 6)

Three variations are described. The choice of method will depend on the indication or goal, and/or the patient's mobility (see Quality criteria, Chapter 2, 4.3, 4.7.7).

The available methods are

— Strokes down the back
— one-handed Einreibung with the patient sitting up
— two-handed Einreibung with the patient lying down (circles with phase shift)

1.1   Strokes down the back

These include spinal or paravertebral strokes and Einreibung of the flanks (see Quality criteria, Chapter 2, 4.4.1, 4.7.7).

1.1.1   Areas of use

— metabolic processes too powerful in the head/neck region (downward)
— hypertension
— help with going to sleep
— beginning and/or conclusion of two-handed back Einreibung lying down

1.1.2   Strokes along the spine

Positioning
The patient lies face down. Depending on the individual situation, feet, abdomen, chest, sternum or head may be supported on small cushions. To relax shoulder and neck muscles, the arms lie beside the head, with upper arms not above shoulder height.

Carer's posture
To begin with it is frontal, one foot forward, with the weight on that leg. Distance from the patient is a bit less than arm's length.

Body and arms move simultaneously during the Einreibung. When the relaxation phase starts, move back a little with the back to make space for the continuing Einreibung. Next take a small step towards the foot end, shifting your weight to the back leg. During the second turning moment come upright and take one step towards the patient's head.

Guideline
Two guidelines run to the left and right of the spine along the longissimus (longest dorsal muscle) from its insertion in the neck region down to the sacrum.

Direction/size
Start at the level of the 7th cervical vertebra and end over the sacrum at the beginning of the gluteal fold.

Both hands are parallel as they move in the caudal direction. The movements may be linear but with the second turning moment coming when in full expansion they should be seen as part of an infinitely great circle.

Distributing the substance
Use as little of the substance as possible, only approximately $^1/_4$ ml (5 drops). Otherwise it will not be possible to increase intensity to optimum level. There is no need for advance distribution over the patient's back, as the small amount just covers the surface of the hand.

Process in the hands
The characteristic feature of this is increasing intensity of contact with local tissue. In the relaxation phase the tissues are taken along a short distance along the guidelines. With more intensive contact, entering in will need more time. Relative to this the relaxation phase needs only slightly more time and is done at a corresponding tempo.

The tissue is subjected to increased intensity of touch by negative pressure of the finger-hand from the metacarpophalangeal joints to the finger pads, without letting the hand slide. When greatest intensity has been reached, tension is relaxed in the whole body but maintained in the finger-hand. Maintain intensity of touch as the hands move down to about the level of the tip of the scapula. Tissue is taken along as far as this and only here does the relaxation stage come in the finger-hand.

You then go with the stream down the back, letting the hands slide lightly to the level of the gluteal fold. Awareness moves from the metacarpophalangeal joints to the finger pads in the process.

In your mind, go with the stream all the way down to the patient's feet. Make the turning moment in the periphery in your thoughts, then take the hands through the air back to the head for the next linear movement.

1.1.3   Lateral strokes

Positioning
As under 1.1.2.

Carer's posture
To begin with, one foot slightly forward, with the weight on the front leg. The position of the hand will be different, so that you bend less than in treating the spine.

Body and arms move simultaneously during the Einreibung.

When letting go of the tension in the hands, take your body back a bit to make space for the continuing Einreibung. Next take a small step towards the foot end, shifting your weight to the back leg. Come upright a little bit after the relaxation phase.

Guideline
For the flank strokes, take your orientation from the median axillary line.

Direction/size
Start posterior to the axillary fold and end at the level of the trochanter. Both hands are parallel as they move in the caudal direction.

Distributing the substance
The flank strokes always follow paravertebral strokes and require no additional substance.

Process in the hands
Give a lot of time to entering locally. Relative to this the relaxation phase needs only slightly more time and is done at a corresponding tempo.

Establish softly sucking contact from the little-finger edge of the palm through the whole mid-hand. After the moment of most intensive contact let go so far in the palms that no tissue will be taken along with the down stroke.

Having let go in outer terms, you again go inwardly with the stream down to the feet, completing the circle by moving through the air until contact is made again at the axillary fold.

1.2   One-handed Einreibung of the back, with the patient sitting up (also known as 'a sitting back') (Plate, Fig. 7)

1.2.1   Areas of use

- Prevention of pneumonia
- to treat respiratory problems, e.g. congestion
- to support upright position after long period of lying down
- tensions
- whole body Einreibung.

1.2.2   Positioning

Sitting up in bed
The patient can sit in his bed by putting his legs at a slight angle, with a knee roll providing support under the thighs. The knees may then go slightly apart. To make the flanks accessible, put a cushion across the knees. Both elbows may then rest on the knees.

Sitting on the edge of the bed
If the feet do not reach the ground, use a footstool or similar to support them. To support the upper body, place cushions on the knees so that the patient is able to sit with forearms crossed in front leaning on the cushions.

On a chair or in a wheelchair
The patient can support himself by resting his arms on the table or the edge of the washbasin (take care to pad cold/hard items of furniture). Another way is to use the back of another chair, with a cushion placed on it.

To keep warm, put a garment on the patient that is open at the back (e.g. dressing gown back to front). Also cover the legs if he is sitting on the edge of the bed. Use a warmed bath towel to cover the whole back, including the hips.

1.2.3   Carer's posture

Without the carer changing sides the Einreibung is done with the same hand for both sides of the back. If you move to the other side of the patient, you'll also change hands. If the patient is sitting on the edge of the bed, you have to change sides and treat always the patient's nearer side.

The body bends more as the movement goes in the caudal direction.

Far side of the back
To treat the far side of the back, stand facing the patient's flank. You will be bending forward more and more as the Einreibung progresses so that the forearm of the hand giving the treatment remains horizontal, at the same time letting your pelvis move back. The hand which you are not using lies on the patient's upper arm on the other side, maintaining continuous contact.

Near side of the back
To treat the side near to you, turn out by an angle of 90 degrees. You will then be shoulder to shoulder with the patient. Again move the pelvis back as the Einreibung goes in the caudal direction.

1.2.4   Guideline/orientation line

The guideline for the down-stroke phase follows the longissimus dorsi muscle.

The enveloping circles do not take their orientation from the direction of muscles. Their boundaries lie between the line of spinous processes and the median axillary line.

1.2.5   Direction/size

Start at the level of the spinous process of the 7th cervical vertebra, ending with the last down stroke over the sacrum. The sizes of the back and of the hand giving the Einreibung determine the size and number of circles (6–8).

The phase of increasing intensity with down strokes of a hand's width goes in the caudal direction. From there the Einreibung continues in a circle taken over the flank, returning to the guideline.

Towards the spine, the form is limited by the longissimus guideline. Up to the tip of the shoulder blade, the circles stay over the shoulder blade. After this, their boundary in the flank is the median axillary line.

1.2.6   Distributing the substance

Put $1/2$–1 ml of the substance (between 10 and 20 drops) in the palm of your hand and distribute down the middle of the side of the back concerned, keeping your touch sliding and moving first from the tip of the shoulder blade to the hips and then from the back of the neck to the hips. The substance will be slowly released from the palm.

1.2.7   Process in the hands

See Quality criteria, Chapter 2; 4.4.5.

Far side of the back
In the phase of increasing intensity, the relaxed palm develops greater intensity by creating suction. This is let go completely with the first turning moment, when contact is also made with the finger-hand. With the circle which follows, contact is evenly relaxed and does not lessen as you return to the guideline.

A help in explaining ongoing awareness through the hand is the image of a clock face. During the phase of increasing intensity (down stroke), from the little-finger edge across the palm to the edge of the thumb. Having inwardly let go, the hand moves in a circle from the spinal column at 9 o-clock to the 5th metacarpophalangeal joint at 6 o-clock, then on to the metacarpophalangeal joint of the middle finger on the flank at 3 o-clock, and the metacarpophalangeal joint of the index finger at 12 o-clock, arriving at the heel of the hand when reaching the spine at 9 o-clock.

Being inwardly relaxed and with ongoing awareness in the planar surface of the hand, we avoid the kind of pressure that would cause tissue to be shifted in the direction of the head and might lead to headaches.

Near side of the back

The two phases and their criteria are the same as for the other side, but the process of ongoing awareness is reversed – mirror image. During the phase of increasing intensity it moves through the finger-hand from edge of little finger to edge of thumb.

During the relaxation phase awareness moves from 3 o-clock at the spine, starting with the final phalanx of the middle finger, reaches the little finger's metacarpophalangeal joint at 6 o-clock, the ball of the thumb/little finger at 9 o-clock, the index finger's metacarpophalangeal joint at 12 o-clock, and the pad of the middle finger again at 3 o-clock.

In the relaxation phase, awareness moves around the whole hand, so that tissue is not displaced, whilst contact remains steady, giving the circle a warming quality.

Conclude with a final intensification over the sacrum. The hand lets go at the first turning moment after intensifying contact in the palm or the finger-hand.

1.3 Two-handed Einreibung, with the patient lying down (also known as the lying back) (Plate, Fig. 8)

Circles with phase shift, intensifying in the flanks.

1.3.1 Areas of use

A few comments first on the special nature of this particular form of Einreibung, with circles in phase shift. The whole makes it possible to transform gravity into levity. It is used when people are particularly subject to gravity (see Quality criteria, Chapter 2; 4.4.6).

Examples

- At the physical level we think of people being bed-bound, so that gravity influences a large body area, especially with paresis, oedema or large areas of coldness in the body.
- Mentally, there may be anxiety states, grieving, exhaustion, tiredness, depression or resignation.
- We find this situation in biography when people lack perspective or have no aims.

1.3.2 Positioning

The Einreibung can only be given to patients who are able to lie face down for some minutes or can be put in a stable position on their side.

Depending on the given situation, head, feet, abdomen, chest or sternum may be supported on small cushions. To relax shoulder and neck muscles, the arms lie beside the head, with upper arms not above shoulder height.

To keep warm, either cover the arms or put a garment on the patient that is open at the back (e.g. dressing gown or jacket back to front). A bath towel covers the whole back.

1.3.3 Carer's posture

The distance from the patient depends on his body size and the carer's reach. It is recommended to give the Einreibung from the right side facing the head of the bed.

Start with one foot slightly forward standing at about the level of the middle thoracic spine. The weight is on the back leg.

1.3.4 Guidelines

The circles on the back do not follow the direction of any muscle. The longissimus as guideline and median axillary line as orientation line merely define the limits.

1.3.5 Direction/size

The whole Rhythmical Einreibung goes in the caudal direction.

The circling movement is anticlockwise. Both hands move in the same direction but are at points in the circle that differ by 180 degrees (phase shift). The right hand starts at 6 o-clock, the left at 12 o-clock, both going towards the flanks. (Plate, Fig. 9)

The upper edges of both circles are at the level of the 7th cervical vertebra, ending at the level of the sacrum. Circles are smallest over the shoulder blades, widening as the Einreibung progresses down the whole left and right back to the sacrum. Circle size varies between shoulders and hips.

1.3.6 Distributing the substance

The area being large, you will need a relatively large amount of substance: 1–1.5 ml (20–30 drops). Distribute it evenly along the sides of the back with an intensity of touch which is like doing relaxed stroking on a water surface.

1.3.7 Process in the hands

The right hand increases intensity as it moves from 6 to 3 o-clock. Awareness goes from finger pads to mid-hand. The left hand increases intensity between 12 and 9 o-clock, with awareness going from heel of hand to mid-hand. After inward relaxation, contact is light for the rest of the circle. With ongoing aware-ness and being inwardly relaxed you avoid your hand getting heavy, which can easily happen on the part of the circle that goes in the cranial direction, the hand being prone (going with gravity).

The right hand increases intensity without additional impulse and entirely in moving contact so that the head will not be burdened. This is a relaxed counterpart to the left hand.

Both hands let intensity go at the first turning moment, the right hand at 3 o-clock, the left at 9 o-clock.

For the moment when the hands meet you have to consider that the patient has already gained an experience of parallel movement, shortly before your hands are at the same height on the flanks.

When a circle is complete, the right hand stays in contact as it moves in the caudal direction, there to start a new circle. The left hand 'jumps' forward from finger-hand to the heel of the hand and can then start the new circle, again at 12 o-clock. Both hands thus shift the start in the caudal direction by one radius.

The Einreibung ends at the same time for both hands. This may be done in two ways:

1   The hands let go at the level of the coccyx – parallel as they follow the guidelines – with contact moving progressively from mid-hand to finger pads.
2   The hands let go in the caudal direction immediately after the first turning moment on the mid-axillary lines – again from mid-hand to finger pads.

2 *Monika Layer* Arm Einreibung

The arm Einreibung is made up of five different part Einreibungen. These are given in the following order:

- hand
- forearm
- elbow
- upper arm
- shoulder

It is usual to treat the whole arm. The shoulder Einreibung is the one most commonly done separately.

2.1 Areas of use

See also Quality criteria, Chapter 2; 4.3.

- help with going to sleep
- stimulation of anabolism, e.g. for cachectic patients with tumours or AIDS
- promoting bodily awareness with hemiplegia
- lymphoedema after mastectomy
- joint pain
- whole body Einreibung.

2.2 Positioning

The patient lies on his back. Cover upper arm and forearm with cloths so that they can be uncovered separately. A long bath towel is good for this. Fix the upper half of it by placing it under the shoulder blade and take it up and forward over the shoulder. Put the lower half under the forearm which lies at an angle, with the hand on the abdomen or chest.

To begin with, place a small roll at the level of the trochanter. Let

1 the forearm rest on this when treating the inner aspect of the upper arm, and
2 the elbow rest on it to give support whilst you treat the shoulder.

Further details concerning positioning are given under the part Einreibungen concerned.

2.3 Carer's posture

The posture changes with the part Einreibungen, and this is described for each in turn.

The arm being highly mobile, good support must be provided or you must keep it securely supported at the elbow and wrist.

The great challenge with an arm Einreibung is to keep the process fluid in spite of several changes in posture. For how this is done, see the 'Taking up and supporting' sections for the part Einreibungen.

2.4 Hand Einreibung (Plate, Fig. 10)

2.4.1 Positioning

The upper arm lies next to the upper body, the forearm is at an angle, with the hand on the abdomen.

2.4.2 Carer's posture

Stand upright though slightly turned to the patient in line with the extended axis of the forearm you are holding. Keep your body relaxed and quiet for this very local Einreibung.

2.4.3 Taking up and supporting

Your flat, supine inner hand takes and supports the patient's hand, your finger-hand stabilizing his wrist. You guide his hand towards your own, placing it on the latter in such a way that the patient's metacarpophalangeal joints lie in the deepest transverse depression in your mid-hand.

The thumb and fingers of carer and patient are on the same side. Put the patient's hand half way between supination and pronation.

When the forearm has been treated after treating the hand, place the hand/forearm on the abdomen again.

2.4.4   Orientation line

This Einreibung does not involve sliding movements of the hands on the tissue. You thus go *with* and not *above* the tissue. The movement is directed towards the middle of the mid-hand as a *site* of orientation.

To get a feeling for the special nature of this Einreibung, call to mind the image of the spiral arrangement of cardiac muscle as it contracts and dilates. Airy kneading imitates the function of cardiac muscle.

2.4.5   Direction/size

The movement goes into the depths of the hand in a spiral and then out again into distant space.

The size depends on the elasticity of the tissue.

2.4.6   Distributing the substance

No distribution as this is a local Einreibung. Sufficient substance is still on your hands after the distribution just made on the forearm.

2.4.7   Process in the hands

Increasing intensity of touch goes in a spiral from the centre of the carer's upper mid-hand to the inner hand of the patient. Ongoing awareness (relative to the patient's hand) moves from 5th finger to wrist. The same happens with the lower hand from 5th finger to finger-hand, following the principle of circles in phase shift (see two-handed strokes down the back, 1.3).

Inner relaxation comes at the moment of most intense contact, without letting go of the tissue under increased intensity of touch. For relaxation, both hands continue in their circles, but now again out and away from the inner part of the hand (away from the bony hand).

When outer relaxation ends, maintain contact, but in your mind take the movement far out. The decision to increase intensity again and therefore change direction towards the inner hand is the 2nd turning moment.

The movement has its centre in the middle of the hand, the rest of the hand merely going along with it. Outwardly it is a very small movement, being done with the tissue and not in the surface area. It does, however, feel like a very large movement.

After the last relaxation phase, the supine patient's hand is placed on the carer's wrist for treating the forearm.

Because of the nearness of the heart, the whole Einreibung is done delicately and with care. Intensity decreases towards the shoulder.

2.5   Forearm Einreibung (Plate, Fig. 11)

2.5.1   Positioning

See under 2.4.

2.5.2   Carer's posture

Stand by the bed, facing the extended axis of the arm to be treated which you have taken up. To ensure that your hand stays close to the arm in best possible flexible adaptation, let it come rather from below. Bend down to do this, and let the pelvis go back in counter movement. Come upright again by bringing the pelvis forward at the end of the relaxation phase.

2.5.3   Taking up and supporting

During the Einreibung, the dorsum of the patient's hand rests on your distal forearm, wrist upon wrist. Your supporting hand is at a downward angle to make room for the hand giving the Einreibung. When the arm has been taken up, check how stable the position is and if necessary make minor corrections in the position of the elbow.

Having treated the patient's hand, treat first of all the ulnar aspect (little finger side) of the forearm, using your inner hand. To change to the radial aspect, your free forearm rolls over, starting from the thumb, to come below the patient's wrist and support it (it is then supine), with the supporting (outer) hand rolling away at the same time.

Taking up and putting down is always done with the flat hand, without any grasping thumb movement. This gives the patient security but also leaves him free, able to release himself from contact at any time.

2.5.4   Guideline

The forearm guidelines pass through the centre of the groups of extensor and flexor muscles of ulna and radius, from wrist to the flexure of the elbow and distal end of the upper arm.

On the forearm, begin the process known as 'playing around the guideline' by letting your hand follow the course of the muscles not in a straight line but diagonally.

2.5.5   Direction/size

The direction of the Einreibung is centripetal, towards the heart. The fingers which have let go are allowed to cross the boundary to the other half of the arm. The circles grow larger in the direction of the elbow, in accordance with the configuration of the forearm.

Concerning the terms 'inside' and 'outside', note that in supination, the continuation of the palm is the 'inside', the continuation of the dorsum of the hand the 'outside' of the forearm. The circles on the ulnar and radial muscle group thus touch both the inside and the outside.

2.5.6   Distributing the substance

Depending on the size of the forearm, distribute $^1/_2$–$^3/_4$ ml (10–15 drops) from wrist to flexure of elbow, following the guidelines.

Contact starts with the pad of the middle finger (mid-line) and follows the guideline towards the mid-hand. As soon as the thickest part of the muscle belly is reached, the hand lets go via the 3rd/2nd/1st phalanx until about a finger's width beyond the flexure of the elbow.

2.5.7   Process in the hands

See also Quality criteria, Chapter 2; 4.7.7.

Increase intensity along the guideline, with the hand palm-down, always starting from the pads of the 2nd and 3rd fingers. You need to work very lightly in this phase, as the touch is coming from above (going with gravity). Increasing contact is sufficient to increase intensity.

Inner relaxation (relaxation in the hand) with change of intention occurs in the place of maximum intensity along the guideline. The change to the supine position follows.

After this, relaxation is in two phases.

1 Contact remaining the same, let the hand change to the supine position, contact growing fuller than it was in the phase of increasing intensity as it is now being made from below.
2 With ongoing contact and ongoing awareness the supine hand lets go all the way to the pad of the third finger.

Supine, the hand works with levity and against gravity. Contact must therefore deliberately be made intense and present, although it is the relaxation phase. Relaxation is then not experienced as an abandoning.

The intention to increase intensity arises when in your mind you let the movement go into the turn out in the periphery, changing the hand's position to prone. The image we may have with increasing intensity and relaxation in a spiral would be 'as if enveloping in clouds'.

Both hands end their movement when after inward relaxation they continue to slide towards the flexure of the elbow, relaxation on contact in the direction of the finger pads until about a finger's width beyond the flexure. Place the patient's hand on his body as described.

2.6   Elbow Einreibung (Plate, Figs 12 & 13)

2.6.1   Positioning

See sections 2.4 and 2.5.

2.6.2   Carer's posture

Stand very close to the bed to allow the hand to move in the axis of the circular route around the elbow joint.

In the phase of increasing intensity, bend forward to allow your hand to make good close contact with the elbow. Come upright again at the end of the relaxation phase.

2.6.3   Taking up and supporting

The outer hand, which has taken up the oil, is supine, supporting the upper arm from outside, whilst the prone inner hand takes the elbow. Place the thumb of that hand against the elbow from inside. Lifting with the thumb and at the same time turning to become supine, the hand receives the elbow with its external epicondyle in the deepest part of the palm. The supporting hand lets the 5th and 4th fingers drop to make room for the hand giving the Einreibung.

Treating a heavy upper arm, let the outer hand hold the elbow and the inner hand use its whole surface to support the upper arm. The patient's forearm thus lies on the carer's forearm.

2.6.4   Orientation line

There is no muscle guideline for the elbow. The orientation line runs right round the joint with all prominent bony structures (epicondyles of upper arm and the head of the ulna) included.

2.6.5   Direction/size

The direction around the joint is determined by the rule that on the arm, intensity is always increased with the hand in prone position. The size depends on the thickness of the patient's arm.

2.6.6   Distributing the substance

The outside hand takes $^1/_2$–$^3/_4$ ml (10–15 drops) for elbow and upper arm, distributing it on the outer and inner aspects of the upper arm before starting to treat the elbow.

No need to use additional substance for the elbow, as this has already been distributed with the first movement and the same movement is repeated several times.

2.6.7   Process in the hands

Increasing intensity starts with the hand prone, from the pad of the 3rd finger via the 2nd and 3rd phalanges towards the mid-hand with ongoing contact and ongoing awareness. Let the hand start on the upper edge of the ulna and increase in intensity until the mid-hand reaches the upper epicondyle.

Now follows inner relaxation by relaxing the hand. The change from being prone to supine begins.

With contact remaining the same, awareness moves from the metacarpophalangeal joint of the 5th finger to that of the 2nd finger, until the mid-hand reaches the lower epicondyle. Let go outwardly by taking the hand back from the mid-hand via the 3rd/2nd/1st phalanx to the starting point. The movement then goes invisibly out far beyond the arm and turns around when the decision comes to repeat. At the same time the hand changes to the prone position.

With the hand's mid-line following the orientation line, create a warm, enveloping roundness around the joint. Though light, contact is intense, with the elbow completely enveloped, and nothing left out.

2.7   Upper arm Einreibung (Plate, Fig. 14)

2.7.1   Positioning

See under Elbow Einreibung, 2.6.

2.7.2   Carer's posture

To treat the outer aspect, move away slightly from the bed, taking a small sideways step. For the inner aspect of the upper arm, stand at an angle of almost 90 degrees (facing the bed).

Move the pelvis back during the phase of increasing intensity, maintaining this posture for the first part of the relaxation phase. Only come upright in the second part until the end of the relaxation phase. Use more counter movement on the inside than on the outside.

2.7.3 Taking up and supporting

To treat the outer aspect after treating the elbow, put the 5th and 4th fingers of the supporting hand on the elbow joint again. Or let the inner hand go back from upper arm to elbow with the help of the outer hand. The finger-hand is lowered during the Einreibung.

The outer hand supports the elbow joint for the inner aspect of the upper arm. Let it roll up from the thumb in such a way that here, too, the epicondyle comes to lie in the deepest part of the palm. At the same time let the inside hand roll away over its thumb. With the inside hand then place the patient's forearm/hand to lie prone on a cushion placed in readiness at about the level of the trochanter. This increases the distance between upper arm and trunk and also the angle in the elbow joint.

Having treated the inner aspect, use your inside hand to place the forearm back on the patients' upper body and cover it. In preparation for treating the shoulder take the upper arm as close as possible to the trunk, supporting the elbow under the towel with your inside hand. The outer hand can then push the cushion under the elbow without meeting resistance. Take care that it lies under the elbow only (not the upper arm), for you do not want to lose any of the free space for treating the shoulder.

2.7.4 Guideline

There are two guidelines on the upper arm. The first, on the outside, runs along the triceps from the head of the ulna to the posterior axillary fold. The other, on the inside, runs along the biceps from the inner flexure of the elbow to the anterior axillary fold.

2.7.5 Direction/size

The local circles done with one hand do not touch the guidelines directly but 'play around them'. The phase of increasing intensity for the circles goes in the direction of the heart.

Outer aspect
The area to be treated is delimited cranially by the deltoid, and caudally by the epicondyle of the humerus. Apart from this the area is the size of the triceps belly.

Inner aspect
The area on the inner aspect is that of the biceps, cranially limited by the lateral margin of the deltoid, caudally by the flexure of the elbow.

The two Einreibungen touch, with no space between, on the superior and inferior aspects of the upper arm.

2.7.6 Distributing the substance

Distribute $^1/_2$–$^3/_4$ ml (10–15 drops) over the outer and inner aspects of the upper arm before treating the elbow. In the outer aspect start from the elbow with the midline of the hand and follow the guideline up to the posterior axillary fold. Build up contact approximately as far as the mid-hand and let go again as far as the finger pads.

On the inner aspect of the upper arm, distribute the substance from the flexure of the elbow via the biceps to the inner margin of the deltoid with short, repeated stroking movements going across the mid-hand.

2.7.7 Process in the hands

See also Quality Criteria, Chapter 2; 4.7.7.

The process in the hand is the same with the inner and outer aspects. The hand is in the prone position, and starting from the finger pads, contact moves towards the mid-hand in the phase of increasing intensity.

Let go inwardly at the moment of maximum contact. Then, changing from the prone to the supine position, let contact remain the same as the hand swings towards the inner margin of the biceps or triceps, so that it can take up the muscle tissue in the mid-hand. Awareness in the mid-hand moves from the fifth to the second finger right across the hand.

From here, take the hand back to the starting point of the circular route, from the third via the second and first phalanges, to arrive at the finger pads in supination.

In your mind, the movement goes invisibly beyond the arm and far into the space behind, where the turn is made. It is only now that your forearm gets to be in prone position.

To conclude the Einreibung, let go inwardly and then allow the finger pads to let go in the direction of the posterior or anterior axillary fold.

On both sides the relaxed fingers touch the hollow between the biceps and triceps muscles on the inner aspect of the upper arm where the brachial artery is (the point where compression is used to stop arterial bleeding). This means that the upper arm is truly enveloped in a way comparable to the way the lower arm is enveloped (in clouds, 2.5).

2.8   Shoulder Einreibung (Plate, Fig. 15)

2.8.1   Areas of use

- Part of arm Einreibung
- Pain with a frozen shoulder

2.8.2   Positioning

With the patient lying down
The arm is in the position described for the end of the upper-arm Einreibung.

As at the beginning of the arm Einreibung, only the head lies on the pillow, leaving the shoulder joints free. A small pillow may be used, or a large one with its corner under the spine at shoulder blade level.

With the patient sitting up
Put a cushion on the patient's lap to support the forearm.

2.8.3   Carer's posture

Shoulder Einreibung with the patient lying down
Your upper arms move parallel to the patient's upper arm, with the lower hand supine and the upper hand in prone position until the turning moment comes. Stand close to the bed for this.

To be able to keep the wrists loose, stand as far away as possible from the shoulder joint and towards the foot end of the bed.

Let your back bend more in the phase of increasing intensity, coming upright a little at the end of the relaxation phase.

Shoulder Einreibung with the patient sitting up
Stand facing the patient's side, so that you can move your hands parallel coming from in front and behind. Your upper body will be bending forward for this.

There is a variation where you work sitting down. The advantage is that you can remain in a relatively upright position.

2.8.4   Guideline/Orientation line

The guideline on the outside of the upper arm goes from the insertion of the deltoid to the tendinous insertion of the muscle at shoulder level. It passes through the middle one of the three parts of the muscle.

During the Einreibung, move freely around the guideline, and in this respect the actual route of the Einreibung is an orientation line. It is oval, in accordance with the form of the deltoid muscle. Anteriorly the oval is limited by the axillary fold. It moves across the acromion in the upper part of the joint, with the posterior axial fold marking the limit towards the back.

2.8.5   Direction/size

The shoulder is enveloped in a 'cap of warmth' using circles with phase shift (see knee and abdominal Einreibung, 4,5.4).

The direction is upwards to shoulder height in front and then moving down again at the back of the shoulder joint. The midlines of the hands follow the orientation line, creating an oval around the shoulder joint that is as large as possible.

The outer hand starts laterally at shoulder height following the circle; at the same time the inner hand starts diagonally to this from the insertion of the deltoid.

2.8.6   Distributing the substance

Distribute about $^1/_4$–$^1/_2$ ml (5 to 10 drops) of the substance over both hands. No need to distribute it over the shoulder joint.

2.8.7   Process in the hands

See also Quality criteria, Chapter 2; 4.7.3, 4.7.7.

Shoulder Einreibung with the patient lying down
The outer hand goes through almost a semicircle – 'Moon hand', the inner hand a full circle – 'Sun hand' (see also 4.7). Your hands are opposite each other and move at the same pace during the phase of increasing intensity.

To increase intensity, the supine outer hand starts with its heel at 11 o'clock (right shoulder) and 1 o'clock (left shoulder) respectively. The inner hand starts prone and with the pads of the three middle fingers at 5 o'clock (right shoulder) and 7 o'clock (left shoulder).

Both hands increase the intensity until the thickest part of the muscle belly is reached at 3 and 9 o'clock respectively. At the same time, awareness has reached the two mid-hands, with contact area and intensity of touch at their greatest.

Then comes the moment when you inwardly let go without losing contact. From now on the two hands work differently. The lower hand does not let the tissue it has received go. After inward relaxation, it completes its movement with awareness moving from mid-hand to finger pads. There the hand lets go.

The upper hand follows the orientation line, crossing the highest point of the joint at the tendinous insertion of the deltoid. At about 2 o'clock (right shoulder) and 10 o'clock (left shoulder) respectively, the finger-hand lets go for a 'dolphin leap' across the top of the shoulder. At 11 o'clock and 1 o'clock respectively it enters in again via the finger pads, completing the circle. Awareness and contact move from the finger pads to the third phalanx, then across the finger-hand and, on the way to the circle's starting point, back to the finger pads.

At the second turning moment, the movement invisibly expands and there turns as the decision is made to continue with another circle. The hand changes direction with this, as you draw your elbow close to the body. At the same time, you make a turn over the finger pad which will not be noticeable to the patient.

In the phase of increasing intensity, let the outer hand receive the tissue as in a bowl, giving your touch correspondingly greater intensity. The inner hand is like the lid on the bowl, its intensity of touch correspondingly less.

In conclusion, the upper hand lets go completely via the finger pads once the circular movement has reached a position at approximately 6 o-clock.

Shoulder Einreibung with the patient sitting up
The process in the hand is the same as when the Einreibung is done with the patient lying down. With the hands approaching from in front and behind, intensity of touch is the same for both.

Conclude over the longissimus dorsi. The anterior hand turns towards the spinal column with its 'dolphin leap'. After increasing contact in the direction of the mid-hand, it lets go until the finger pads are reached. The hand then lies over the longissimus with the fingers pointing in the caudal direction.

3   *Monika Layer*   Chest Einreibung (Plate, Figs 16 & 17)

3.1   Areas of use

See also Quality criteria, Chapter 2; 4.3

* Respiratory problems
* Treatment of bronchitis
* Post-operative pain, e.g. after mastectomy
* Prevention of pneumonia
* Whole body Einreibung

3.2   Positioning

The patient is lying flat on his back, or with the chest area slightly raised if there are breathing difficulties, his head not too deep down in the pillows. His arms are beside his body at an adequate distance. A knee roll under the knees serves to relax the abdominal wall. Ask the patient to turn his head to the other side from where the procedure is being done.

3.3   Carer's posture

Stand to the right of the bed, one leg forward a bit, facing the bed. Essentially the weight is on the back leg.

Use the same hand to do the Einreibung on both sides of the body, remaining in the same place. Start on the side further away from you. To change to the near side, take a small step towards the foot end. Otherwise maintain the same position throughout.

Come upright a little before the second phase of increasing intensity. The direction in your hand rotates by 90 degrees as you move to the flank. Move back slightly in the pelvis as contact increases in the course of this movement.

Let your free hand rest laterally on the origin of the deltoid on the near side. As you proceed, develop an inner 'listening' relationship between the two hands.

The Einreibung may also be done with the patient sitting up. In this case, you will need to change position and hands.

3.4   Orientation line

No muscles serve to give the Einreibung definite direction in the chest region, nor do the functions of heart and lung. Take your orientation from the anatomical structures described below.

3.5   Direction/size

In your mind, the Einreibung is a large circle going from the clavicle to the tip of the sternum and then out to the flank. When the hand has let go, complete the circle in the air, going back to the clavicle.

The limits are set cranially by the clavicle, and towards the mid-body by the sternum. The lower costal arch marks the caudal, and the median axillary line the lateral limit.

3.6   Distributing the substance

Distribute the $^1/_2$–$^3/_4$ ml (10 to 15 drops) as you proceed with the Einreibung.

3.7   Process in the hands

See also Quality criteria, Chapter 2; 4.7.7.

Two rhythms are on top of each other with a chest Einreibung. The larger one characteristically comes with the movement from below the clavicle to the tip of the sternum and from there to the flank or median axillary line.

The two phases are further differentiated in themselves by increasing and decreasing contact. Half-way to the tip of the sternum, contact increases until awareness has reached the mid-hand. After this contact decreases towards the tip of the sternum until only the pad of the middle finger is still in contact.

The second route is also differentiated in

itself. Starting from the finger pads, let the hand lie flat as it follows the costal arches until it reaches the median axillary line. Half-way along – depending on the size of your hand – it may be that the whole hand is in contact; at the median axillary line, only the finger-hand is in touch. Going towards the flank, let the intensity of touch increase, although this is the relaxation phase.

Finish by taking the hand away flatly from the middle of the finger-hand. Complete the form by returning along a circular path in the air to the starting point below the clavicle.

Inner relaxation and ongoing awareness help you to differentiate the two rhythms and maintain the quality of lightness although the hand is largely in the prone position.

4   *Monika Layer*   Abdominal Einreibung (Plate, Fig. 18)

4.1   Areas of use

- To stimulate peristalsis and overcome constipation
- flatulence
- intestinal spasms
- whole body Einreibung.

4.2   Positioning

The patient lies flat on his back, or with the upper body slightly raised. Arms at the sides, slightly away from the body. Hands may be placed on the chest.

Place a warm towel or cloth around the abdomen so that it may be opened at the front. Having taken up the substance, open the cloth and let its ends cover the flanks closely so that the kidney region will not get cold. Put a roll under the knees to relax the abdominal wall.

4.3   Carer's posture

Stand to the right of the patient and close to the bed, without leaning on it. Depending on the height of the bed and your own height, bend down as required, standing at a suitable distance towards the foot end. During the phase of increasing intensity, let your pelvis go back, coming slightly upright again at the end of the relaxation phase.

Let your hand lie flat on the abdomen, with your lower arms at the same level. You are looking at the area to be treated from the direction of the legs, with the patient's head at the upper limit of your field of vision.

4.4   Orientation line

Our orientation line in the abdominal region is a circle which does not fit in with the form of any organ. We choose this form because the non-specific round encompasses the many different abdominal organs, and the circular movement made with two hands has very much a warming effect.

Over the colon, the descending colon provides an orientation line.

4.5   Direction/size

The direction of the circular Einreibung takes its orientation from the colon. It goes clockwise, therefore. The stroke follows the descending colon from the left colic flexure to the inguinal region.

The size of the circle is determined by the bony structures – left and right iliac crests, left and right costal arches and the two pubic bones. The circle itself is the largest possible between costal arches and edges of iliac bones.

4.6   Distributing the substance

Let approximately $^3/_4$–1 ml (15–20 drops) of the substance warm up well in your hands. Coming from the direction of the flanks make contact with both hands at the height of the navel, your fingers pointing towards the cranium. Let your hands move along the orientation line towards the navel without increasing in intensity until they are at 3 and 9 o'clock. Continue clockwise from there (description continued for relaxation phase).

4.7   Process in the hands

See also Quality criteria, Chapter 2; 4.4.6, 4.7.3, 4.7.7.

Both hands move simultaneously in circles with phase shift (see also Knee Einreibung, 5.4). The left hand moves in a full circle ('Sun hand'), the right almost a semicircle ('Moon hand'). Let the touch generally have a quality of lightness. See the abdomen as a sphere in your mind to avoid working as though on a flat surface.

Right hand. Starting from the heel of the hand, the right hand enters on the left (the patient's left) from the solar plexus (1 o'clock), developing contact until the mid-hand is at about navel height (3 o'clock). Following the turning moment, it lets go via the 3rd, 2nd and 1st phalanges until it lets go completely at the finger pads within the pelvic crest to the left of the bladder region (5 o'clock).

Left hand. The lateral side of the 5th finger enters in the region of the appendix, to the right of the bladder. It moves in the cranial direction within the pelvic crest via the metacarpophalangeal joint of the fifth finger until it has developed the most intensive contact at navel height, at the same time as the right hand. Awareness now lies in the mid-hand.

After the first turning moment, awareness moves from mid-hand towards the heel of the hand. With this, let go with the pads of the third/fourth/fifth fingers to the right of the solar plexus so that the hand 'leaps' across the plexus. The distal phalanges of the second to fifth fingers make contact again to the left of the solar plexus. With increasing and decreasing contact and awareness at the same time moving across the finger-hand, the hand moves in the caudal direction within the pelvic crest until the distal phalanges reach the bladder region (at 5 o'clock). Another leap, this time to cross the bladder region. The next circle then begins, again with the lateral side of the fifth finger.

Over the descending colon the movement, or the hand in question, has a bit more of an accent, to give emphasis in the direction of the anus. The left hand thus uses the increase in contact during the relaxation phase to apply more intensive touch to the tissues again over the descending colon.

This part of the abdominal Einreibung ends with the relaxation phase of the left hand being taken to its conclusion – before the second turning moment on the left before the bladder region.

4.7.1   Colon strokes

See also Quality criteria, Chapter 2; 4.7.7.

This concludes the abdominal Einreibung.

Increase intensity with the right hand, placing it over the right flexure, with the fingers pointing to the spine. Make contact going from the edge of the little finger to the thumb, taking up the tissue in the direction of the ceiling. As soon as the mid-hand has reached maximum intensity, let go inwardly and then let the stroke move towards the groin. Awareness jumps to the heel of the hand with this and then moves from the mid-hand to the pad of the third finger. There the hand lets go completely. Let your left hand maintain contact in the right flank during this, 'listening' to the right hand's activity as this repeatedly takes the same route.

5   *Monika Layer*   Leg Einreibung

Depending on the situation or indication, different part leg Einreibungen may be used individually or in combination. A leg Einreibung includes treating the lower leg, knee, thigh and foot (see also Quality criteria, Chapter 2; 4.3).

5.1   Areas of use

- Prevention of thrombosis
- Prevention of pressure ulcers
- Circulatory problems in the legs
- Cold extremities
- Pain in the region of the lower leg and knee (arthritis, rheumatism, trauma)
- Whole body Einreibung

5.2   Contraindications

- Thrombosis
- Open wounds

Please note
In pregnancy, leg Einreibungen should only be done by experienced hands; a danger of miscarriage exists especially in the first trimester.

5.3   Lower leg Einreibung (Plate, Fig. 19)

5.3.1   Areas of use

- As part of a leg or whole-body Einreibung
- Combined with foot Einreibung to help induce sleep
- Calming anxieties
- Harmonizing the breathing, especially if there are problems with exhalation (asthma)
- Prevention of thrombosis

5.3.2   Positioning

Using a knee roll, position the leg so that the hollow of the knee is free for two finger widths in the direction of the thigh. The distance from the bed should be sufficient to allow your hand adequate freedom of movement. Marked external rotation can be balanced out by supporting the hip or adjusting the knee roll, but need not be cancelled out completely.

5.3.3   Carer's posture

Stand with one leg forward and facing at a distance which will allow your lower arms to move parallel to the lower leg. In the phase of increased intensity, shift your weight back a little, making your back more rounded. Come upright a little more at the end of the relaxation phase, when your lower arm is taken back to the body again.

Let your free hand lie on the outside, at maximus muscle level, with the fingers in the cranial direction. On the inside it can either hold the heel in its palm or lie against the inside of the ankle. In either case it should not impede the active hand, and you should feel no constriction in the chest.

5.3.4   Guidelines

All four leg guidelines start at the heel, running together along the Achilles tendon. They divide into two on the lower leg where the gastrocnemius divides. They run straight, merely following the sculptured form of the muscle in the direction of the muscle insertions on the femur (3rd and 4th guideline, see 5.5.4).

5.3.5   Direction/size

The direction of the circles is centripetal and towards the heart.

The circles start on the guideline, swinging outwards towards the tibia and back to the guideline, progressing towards the knee in spirals. The circles on either side thus run in opposite directions.

The size of the circles depends on the width

of the Achilles tendon, the increase in connective tissue and the thickness of the muscle belly.

5.3.6   Distributing the substance

Use one supine hand after the other to distribute $1/2$–1 ml of the substance, following the guideline with the midline of the hand.

Make first contact with the finger pad on the heel-bone. Increase contact steadily up to the thickest part of the muscle, then letting go again by a fairly short route towards the back of the knee with the metacarpophalangeal joint of the index finger.

5.3.7   Process in the hands

Increase intensity with the hand supine each time, i.e. in opposition to gravity.

It is not possible to swing sideways and change to the prone position when over the Achilles tendon. Yet the process of letting go inwardly and the change in intention – in terms of receiving and giving – lead to a change in quality. The short route is from finger pad to second phalanx and back again.

As the circles grow larger, maintain contact at the same level in the upper third of the circle, having let go inwardly, and decrease it continually on returning to the guideline. Do the second turning moment – even with the smallest circles – by letting the movement go beyond your arm in your thoughts and turn when out in the distance.

Conclude with the relaxation phase of the last circle. This goes towards the back of the knee, about two finger widths beyond the crease at the knee. The movement is given over in the cranial direction, as the guideline stream continues on.

5.4   Knee Einreibung (Plate, Fig. 20)

5.4.1   Areas of use

* Pain in the knee
* Trauma with swelling

* Cold knees
* Part of whole body, thigh or leg Einreibung

5.4.2   Positioning

With the Einreibung given on its own, place a roll directly under the knee. If a thigh Einreibung follows, see under 5.5.

5.4.3   Carer's posture

Stand facing the patient's head, one foot forward, and far enough away to be able to use both arms freely and maintain a flexible equilibrium. Have your forearms parallel to the lower leg.

The body's centre of gravity is in the pelvis. The weight rests mainly on the back leg.

In the phase of increased intensity, take the pelvis back and let your form be more rounded. Come upright a little at the end of the relaxation phase.

5.4.4   Guidelines/orientation lines

The knee is mainly tendons and ligaments all round, though these do not circle the joint. We therefore look for guidelines and orientation lines.

One guideline for the knee joint is on the medial aspect – the course of the sartorius from tibia to articular cleft. The second guideline follows the tensor fasciae latae which is tangential to the joint on the lateral aspect at the level of the articular cleft.

The continuation of this, going in a circle around the knee joint, should be seen as an orientation line. In the upper part of the knee, the tendon of the rectus femoris is at right angles to the direction taken with the Einreibung.

5.4.5   Direction/size

Use both hands at the same time in circles with phase shift. The direction is from below/inner to above/outer. The inner hand makes a full circle (Sun hand), the outer hand only a semicircle (Moon hand). This form envelops the whole joint.

The circles are the same size throughout, as determined by guideline and orientation line.

The point of first contact for the inner hand arises from the point of insertion for the sartorius. The outer hand starts on the lateral aspect of the knee joint, outside the rectus femoris.

5.4.6   Distributing the substance

$^1/_4$-$^1/_2$ ml (5 to 10 drops) as a guide. Distribute this directly with both hands as you do the Einreibung.

5.4.7   Process in the hands

See also Quality criteria, Chapter 2; 4.4.6, 4.7.3.

Increase intensity using both hands at the same time. The inner hand begins with the pads of the middle three fingers, the outer hand with the heel of the hand. Along that short route, awareness in both hands goes as far as the mid-hand.

Starting point for the left leg: The inside hand starts at 7 o'clock, the outside hand at 1 o'clock.

Starting point for the right leg: The inside hand starts at 5 o'clock, the outside hand at 11 o'clock.

When they are opposite at 3 and 9 o'clock, both mid-hands are over the articular space. After the moment of most intense contact they go into the process of inwardly letting go at the first turning moment.

The inside hand makes a 'dolphin leap' across the rectus femoris. Attention first moves from mid-hand to heel of hand. It then 'leaps' to the finger pads and until the articular space is reached moves to the metacarpophalangeal joints and then back to the finger pads again.

The second turning moment comes when in your mind the movement goes beyond your arm and turns when out in the periphery at the same time adducting the elbow as you make the turn over the pad of the middle finger.

The outer hand lets go of the knee joint via the finger pads (right leg, 7 o'clock; left leg, 5 o'clock). It completes the circle as it moves

through the air if there is to be a further phase of increased intensity.

Both hands envelop the knee by recreating its spherical form, always inwardly relaxed, with ongoing awareness and observing the counter movements.

Conclude the knee Einreibung either

- by continuing on into a thigh Einreibung, or
- by letting go with the inside hand
  a) on completion of the relaxation phase (warmth aspect) or
  b) letting it go along the guideline of the sartorius after the first turning moment, doing so in the direction of the finger pads (flowing stream aspect).

5.5   Thigh Einreibung (Plate, Fig. 21)

5.5.1   Areas of use

- As part of a leg or whole-body Einreibung
- To stimulate digestion

The thigh relates closely to the system of metabolism and limbs. A Rhythmical Einreibung will therefore stimulate digestion.

5.5.2   Positioning

Put a roll under the outside of the knee and towards the lower leg so that the thigh is slightly elevated, allowing easy access to the outside of the thigh. Put something under the heel of the foot to reduce pressure on the calf muscle.

5.5.3   Carer's posture

Stand with one foot slightly forward, facing the head of the bed. The distance is such that your forearms can move parallel to the thigh without blocking the outside arm for yourself.

Shift your weight back a little, rounding your form more, in the phase of increased intensity, and come upright a bit again at the end of the relaxation phase.

The length of the thigh makes it necessary to change position as you do the Einreibung, moving in the cranial direction in steps of a hand's width.

5.5.4   Guidelines

The two guidelines for the thigh Einreibung are

- the tendon of the tensor fasciae latae (line of trouser seam) from the outer edge of the tibia to the pelvic crest, and
- the course of the sartorius from the inner edge of the tibia to the pelvic crest along the inner margin of the quadriceps. This guideline delimits the inguinal venous triangle where no impulse should be given to avoid congestion.

5.5.5   Direction/size

Starting from the knee Einreibung, use circles with phase shift, taking them in the same direction. The shape of the thigh is such that the circles will usually get larger at first and then smaller than they were on the knee. The two guidelines limit them and cause them to move sideways as you move towards the hip joint.

5.5.6   Distributing the substance

Distribute the $^1/_2$–$^3/_4$ ml (12 to 15 drops) required with both hands simultaneously. Let the inside hand follow the sartorius, increasing and then reducing contact. Let the outside hand start lateral to the knee, its midline following the tensor fasciae latae, again with contact increasing and then decreasing.

Let both hands make first contact with the pads of the middle fingers, letting go again with the pads of the middle fingers in the region of the trochanter. The inside hand increasingly assumes the prone position, resulting in progressively less intensity of touch compared to the outside hand which remains supine.

5.5.7   Process in the hands

Increase intensity using the inside hand along the short distance of the sartorius guideline. At the same time use the outside hand to increase intensity on the tensor fasciae latae.

The route for increasing intensity is relatively short, as it is entirely on the guidelines. The inside hand becomes progressively more prone as you move towards the hip. Cross the quadriceps with a great 'dolphin leap'.

In the phase of increased intensity the outside hand becomes supine, and the relaxed finger-hand makes contact with the guidelines on the underside of the thigh. As a result, the thigh is truly enveloped.

At the end/high point of the phase of increased intensity both mid-hands are on the guidelines and opposite to one another – in line with the articular space on the knee.

Finer detail

Use the inside hand to increase intensity over a short distance along the sartorius guideline, with awareness moving from the pad of the middle finger to the mid-hand.

At the same time let the outside hand increase intensity along the tensor fasciae latae.

Having inwardly let go at the first turning moment, awareness in the inside hand moves to the heel of the hand. The 'dolphin leap' goes across the quadriceps. Let the hand then swing via the finger-hand to the pads of the fingers on the outside of the thigh, thus returning to the guideline with contact steadily getting less. The second turning moment comes shortly before the sartorius. Along a short distance of the tensor fasciae latae the outside hand increases intensity from heel to mid-hand. After the first turning moment, it lets go of contact via the pads of the fingers, completes the circles as it moves through the air, and enters again opposite to the inside hand.

In addition to ongoing awareness, inner relaxation and the counter movements ensure that the inside hand in particular can be sufficiently light.

Conclude the Einreibung in the region of the trochanter by letting go with both hands. Let the outside hand take its usual route. Let the inside hand go from mid-hand to finger pads after the first turning moment, letting the movement go in the cranial direction.

5.6   Foot Einreibung

5.6.1   Areas of use

See also Quality criteria, Chapter 2; 4.3.

- Whole body
- Cold feet
- Conclusion of leg Einreibung
- Superficial breathing in spasms
- To 'earth' people who are not wholly 'together'
- Bringing down away from the head
- To help with going to sleep, possibly in combination with a lower leg Einreibung.

5.6.2   Forms

A simple foot Einreibung is made up of four forms:

1   two-handed strokes
2   heel circles
3   ankle circles
4   strokes on the soles

5.6.3   Positioning

The patient lies on his back for all forms. If the foot end of the bed gets in the way you might find it easier to reach the foot if you elevate the mattress with a pillow put underneath and position the leg to face slightly outwards. Support the knee with a roll.

5.6.4   Two-handed strokes (Plate, Fig. 22)

Carer's posture
Bending in a relaxed way and in dynamic balance, one foot forward and feet slightly apart, facing the bed. Having concluded the phase of increased intensity come upright by moving the pelvis forward or towards the foot under treatment.

Orientation line
On the dorsum of the foot, the line runs down the middle from the proximal end of the metatarsus to the distal phalanges of the toes. The guideline on the sole is opposite to this.

Direction
Use both hands, going from arch to toes.

Distributing the substance
There is no need to do this separately. Use as little as possible to get good contact (c. $\frac{1}{4}$ ml, or 4 to 6 drops).

Process in the hands
See also Quality criteria, Chapter 2; 4.7.3, 4.7.7.

First make contact with the lower hand by softly fitting the ball of the thumb into the arch. Then make contact with the middle of the base of the upper hand on the highest point of the dorsum. As the stroke is made, let the second and third fingers of the upper hand slide to the inside of the foot. This will enable you to envelop the toes fully.

Contact with the lower hand is at the same intensity – the way the sole of the foot progressively changes contact when walking – whilst the upper hand merely follows and envelops.

Decreasing contact in the distal direction corresponds to the relaxation phase, although the intensity of touch maintains the same intensity to the end of the stroke.

In the course of the stroke, awareness in the upper hand moves to the finger pads, awareness in the lower hand to the edge of the index finger.

5.6.5   Heel circles (Plate, Fig. 23)

Carer's posture
Stand with one foot ahead of the other facing the bed. Bend greatly during the phase of increased intensity, coming completely upright in the relaxation phase. Let the palm of your free hand support the lower leg above the Achilles tendon.

Orientation line
This circles the heel, starting at the inside of the calcaneus and going like the thong of a sandal

across the Achilles tendon, returning to its starting point below the outside of the malleolus and along the heel part of the sole.

Direction/size
The circle swings around the heel from the inner to the outer aspect of the foot and then back again (right foot anticlockwise, left foot clockwise).

The size depends on the foot in question. It should go completely round the heel, not touching the malleolus.

Distributing the substance
There is no need to do this specially.

Process in the hands
Start with increasing intensity on the inner 'sandal thong' using the pads of the three middle fingers. As the hand continues to envelop the heel, it recreates its form, fitting itself closely to the heel. The moment of greatest intensity has come when the heel lies in your mid-hand and this has taken the weight of the lower leg. The hand is supine at this point.

In the relaxation phase along the outside and sole of the heel, awareness moves from palm to finger pads. Contact remains close, although very light, so that the hand does not tickle.

The second turning moment is when inwardly out in the distance, at the same time rotating over the pad of the middle finger.

5.6.6 Ankle circles (Plate, Fig. 24)

Carer's posture
Stand facing the sole of the foot, bending considerably in the phase of increased intensity, your forearms being at the level of the foot. Come upright at the end of the relaxation phase, widening your shoulder girdle.

Orientation line
On the inner and outer aspects of the foot, two orientation lines play around the ankle joint in a circle. They go from the left and right of the Achilles tendon to the dorsum of the foot. There they run parallel to below the ankle, returning to the starting point at the Achilles tendon in a semicircle.

Direction/size
The circles go from below (Achilles tendon) upwards (towards the dorsum).

The size depends on the ankle joint. The Einreibung moves around it loosely but in a closely defined form.

Distributing the substance
There is no need to do this specially.

Process in the hands
See also Quality criteria, Chapter 2; 4.4.6, 4.7.7.

Only the finger-hands are in contact with this Einreibung. The distal phalanges of the second to fourth fingers move around the ankles, the thumbs lying lightly on the dorsum.

Increase intensity as you move from Achilles tendon to dorsum, with the hands changing from being supine to prone. The tissue is taken up successively by the phalanges. Having inwardly let go, let the pads of the index, middle and ring fingers take the tissue subject to increased intensity along with a clear impulse in the distal direction (towards the toes). Relax the intensity by bending the fingers during the stroke, letting them move towards the thumb.

In the second part of the relaxation phase, let the finger pads slide back to the starting point without impulse, the hand being prone.

5.6.7 Strokes on the sole of the foot (Plate, Figs 25 & 26)

Carer's posture
Stand at the side of the bed, facing the outside of the foot. Bend down well, taking back your pelvis, so that the forearm of the hand doing the strokes can be horizontal.

The free hand warmly envelops, lying lightly and horizontally across the dorsum.

Orientation line
This originates in the transverse vault under the second metatarsal joint, at the lowest point

between the eminences. It runs straight from there across the arch to the heel.

Direction/size
The direction follows the orientation line from the toes to the end of the heel. Size is determined by the foot.

Distributing the substance
There is no need to do this specially.

Process in the hands
See also Quality criteria, Chapter 2; 4.7.7.

The softest part of the ball of the thumb makes contact in the deepest part of the transverse arch like in a 'press stud system', at the same time using slight torque and increasing intensity on the inner foot. This is intensive local contact, which at the same time also has a suction quality. Relax inwardly, but as with strokes parallel to the spine in such a way that the tissue subject to increased intensity is gently taken along for the first part of the relaxation phase. The ball of the thumb slides to the heel, getting lighter as the hand assumes the prone position. Awareness moves in a circle around the ball of the thumb and towards the back of the hand. When the hand has let go, continue the movement going out inwardly into the distance.

Sources
Grosse-Brauckmann E. personal unpublished notes and scripts from her teaching in 1990–2001.

Layer M. unpublished notes and scripts from teaching and workshops 1990–2001.

6   *Rolf Heine*   The pentagram Einreibung

6.1   Background

The pentagram is the second basic form used in Rhythmical Massage, the first being the lemniscate [Hauschka 1972]. The latter is used in many variations in Rhythmical Einreibungen, but there is no established form for the pentagram. One way of making the five-pointed star your basic form is to divide a whole-body Einreibung into five part Einreibungen of the back and limbs, doing them on consecutive days.

The form of pentagram Einreibung presented here takes about 10 minutes. It was developed when working with two seriously ill young patients at the Filder Clinic in Germany and from 1990 onwards has proved effective in treating many patients.

It differs from a classic Rhythmical Einreibung in that it is limited to five very small skin areas. This reduction in outer movement demands increased sensitivity in the hands, something which the pentagram Einreibung has in common with organ Einreibungen. Like these, the pentagram Einreibung acts on the whole organism. Unlike organ Einreibungen, the position of the treated areas relates not to a physical organ (e.g. the kidney) but the functional relationship between the body's centre and periphery (heart and capillaries). Just as centre and periphery are rhythmically linked by the circulation, so does the human being live in the rhythm of self-awareness when awake, and forgetfulness of self in sleep; between living experience of self in sensory perception and shaping the world in doing; between connecting with the living body (incarnation) and letting go of the living body (excarnation). The pentagram Einreibung influences these particular rhythms, bringing them into balance. It is an instrument for nursing care and therapy when one-sided tendencies develop in the sphere of the physical body or of soul and spirit.

6.1.1   The five-pointed star and the human form

If an adult human being stands upright, legs apart and with his arms raised to about the level of the diaphragm, the form that results is a regular five-pointed star (pentagram). This has been the occult sign for the human being from antiquity. (Fig. 3.1) The therapeutic use of the five-pointed star is not, however, based on symbolism, but on the mathematical and organic principle which pentagram and human form have in common, and that is the Golden Section.

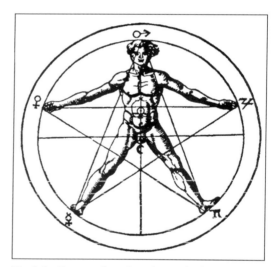

Fig. 3.1   Drawing based on the work of Agrippa von Nettesheim (16th c.).

6.1.2   The Golden Section

The Golden Section is a relative proportion that has been used in art and architecture for millennia. Buildings, interiors, paintings and sculptures feel particularly harmonious to those who see them if their forms show the proportions of the Golden Section.

The Golden Section divides a distance in such a way that the shorter part m relates to the greater part M as the greater part does to the whole (m + M). Put in a mathematical formula this is

$$m : M = M : (m + M)$$

If you divide a line which is 10 cm long according to the Golden Section, the shorter distance, the 'minor', will be 3.72 cm, the longer distance, the 'major', 6.18 cm. To determine the major for a line of any length, you therefore merely have to multiply the total length by 0.618.

The Golden Section thus expresses ancient wisdom in mathematical terms: 'The whole relates to the greater as the greater does to the lesser.' The cosmos (the whole) relates to the earth (the major) as the earth does to the human being (the lesser). Man is the microcosm!

6.1.3   The Golden Section in the human form

In the adult human form, almost all proportions show the Golden Section relationship. This remarkable fact is demonstrable on the skeleton and also the ideal form (Fig. 3.2).

This can be illustrated by looking at some of the main proportions. The whole form, measured from the top of the head to the soles of the feet, divides at waist level in Golden Section proportions, giving us the upper and the lower body. The upper body shows the Golden Section from waist to base of neck (major) and base of neck to occiput (minor). The lower body is divided in Golden Section proportions below the knee. Characteristically, people like to emphasize the harmonious proportions of the body at the waist, base of neck and the narrowing below the knee by wearing belts or decorating the neckline or hem of a skirt.

The Golden Section proportions are found only in the adult form. A child's body still has proportions of a different kind and will only come close to the 'ideal' proportion of the Golden Section after further growth.

The human form thus develops towards an ideal, and it appears that the Golden Section is the morphogenetic principle behind human growth.

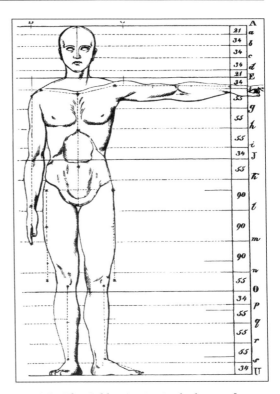

Fig. 3.2   The Golden Section in the human form.

6.1.4   The Golden Section in the pentagram

Mention has already been made of the outward relationship between human being and pentagram. But is there also an inner relationship between the geometrical figure and the human form? Looking at a regular five-pointed star we find that all the intersections show the proportions of the Golden Section (Fig. 3.3). The

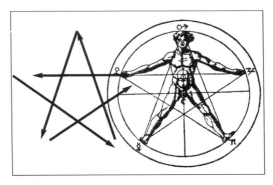

Fig. 3.3   The route taken to develop the pentagram.

pentagram thus is not only a striking symbol for the human being but also an exact mathematical description of the ideal human form.

6.1.5   The pentagram and the human ether body

Rudolf Steiner called the energy composition which organizes the physical body the body of creative powers or ether body. Ultimately this organizes all growth and regenerative processes. It makes up the energy composition which in life is present throughout the physical body and maintains its form. At death, the ether body separates from the physical body which then decomposes, i.e. loses its form.

The Golden Section has been identified as the morphological development goal for the human form. It is thus an essential structure in the body of creative powers, and we can understand why Rudolf Steiner called the pentagram, also constituted on the basis of the Golden Section, 'the skeleton of the ether body'.

6.2   Technique for the pentagram Einreibung

The Einreibung follows the way in which the five-pointed star evolves on the human form (Fig. 3.4). It is given on the forehead, forearms and lower legs.

6.2.1   Practical details

Preparation

- Materials
  - Ointment or oil, as indicated
- Informing the patient about
  - the aims of the treatment (to harmonize, calm),
  - time required (*c.* 10 minutes, plus 30 minutes rest),
  - modalities (no distractions during the treatment and rest period — talking, visitors, reading, etc.)
- Preparing the patient
  - Let him go to the toilet

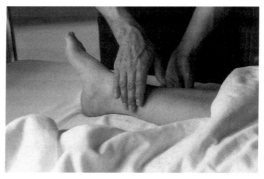

Fig. 3.4   Technique on right lower leg.

- See that he is lying comfortably on his back
- Take off bracelet or wristwatch
- Take off stockings or tights
- Cover the patient up to the chest
- Place arms on top of the covers, parallel to the upper body, folding the covers back over the forearms
- Preparing the room
  - Air the room before giving the Einreibung, then close the window
  - Push the bed far enough away from the wall to allow you to walk freely around it
  - Switch off the telephone
- Carer's preparations
  - Make sure of a calm mind, and warm hands
  - Apply a pea-sized amount of ointment to the back of one hand. (Serves as a reservoir during the procedure to avoid having to reach for the ointment tube several times. – If oil is used, it will however be necessary to reach for the bottle a number of times.)

Method

- Stand to the right side of the patient at the level of his head.
- Spread a little ointment or oil on the pads of the index, middle and ring finger of your right hand.
- Let the left hand be awake, though it does not touch the patient.
- Bring the right hand on the patient's forehead, touching an area of approximately

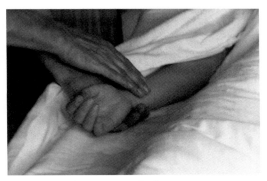

Fig. 3.5 Technique on right forearm.

2.5 cm diameter above the root of the nose, doing so as gently as possible.

- Make 5 or so small, almost stationary, anticlockwise circles in this area.
- Let the hand come away as gently as it first made contact.
- Come upright and move to the level of the right foot.
- Uncover the right foot and the distal lower leg.
- Put a little ointment or oil on your finger pads again.
- Treat an area of approximately 2.5 cm diameter about three finger widths above the inside of the ankle immediately below the tibia, making 7–10 circles of the kind described for the forehead. The left hand again does not touch the patient.
- Cover the lower leg and foot again.
- Come upright and go round the foot end to the left side of the bed to stand at the level of the patient's forearm.
- Uncover the left forearm.
- Put a little ointment or oil again on your finger pads.
- Treat an area about two finger widths proximal to the heel of the hand in the same way as described for the lower leg, with c. 7 circles, which now run clockwise, however.
- Place the forearm and hand on the bedcover again and cover by folding this over from the outside.
- Stand up straight and walk round the head end of the bed to the right forearm.
- Treat the right forearm the same way as the left, but anticlockwise.

- Stand straight again and walk past the foot end of the bed to the left lower leg.
- Treat the left lower leg like the right one, but with clockwise circles.
- Stand up straight and walk past the head end of the bed to the starting point which is to the right of the head.
- Treat the forehead once more with 1–3 circles.
- In conclusion let the right hand touch the bedcovers in the patient's heart region. Use only the slightest pressure.

Rest and follow-up

- The patient should rest for at least 30 minutes.
- If possible and appropriate, talk to the patient about sensations and moods experienced during the Einreibung. Important images and thoughts will often have come up, and one should make time for a talk when occasion arises.

6.2.2 Rationale for and deepening of the technique

Some frequently asked questions will be considered below.

Why do you treat the pulse region of forearms and lower legs rather than the palms of the hand and inner aspects of the feet?

Wrists and ankles are particularly temperature-sensitive zones. These are the areas which determine if hands and feet will warm up. People who tend to suffer from cold hands and feet will be able to confirm that wristlets are often the only way of dealing with the situation.

In the pulse regions, the heart beat shows itself in the body periphery. This may serve as another indication for it being the right choice of site.

Ultimately, many different trials applying Einreibungen to the palm and/or forearm have shown that the effect is by far the greatest in the location described.

Why do you treat the forehead?

It is the place on the body surface where the body temperature is reflected in the most constant way. If the rectal temperature is 37°C, the temperature on the forehead will be approx. 34°C. With a raised temperature it will go up in proportion to the core temperature. This is not the case in the extremities. A reliable qualitative assessment of the temperature can therefore only be gained on the forehead.

Thus the forehead, wrists and ankles each show a different special relationship to the human warmth organism. On the forehead, the internal temperature shows itself on the outside; in the wrists and ankles the organism regulates its temperature conditions in relation to the environment.

Why is contact pointwise and not planar?
Experience has shown that pointwise touch with stationary circles leads to intense concentration of the mind. This effect is lost if you treat a larger area.

Why the touch over the heart after the Einreibung?
With the pentagram Einreibung, the patient's body is merely touched with the finger pads in its periphery. As a result, conscious awareness shifts wholly to the outer boundaries of the body. The very light touch over the heart lets the patient come to himself again. It puts the accent on rhythmical alternation between opening up to the outside and return to the body, between inhalation and exhalation, arterial and venous blood, and between incarnation and excarnation. Patients will sometimes manage to make this rhythmical movement on their own, without the touch to the heart.

How many circles should be made in the different locations?
The forehead is the site most sensitive to touch with the pentagram Einreibung. The first time, 5 to 7 circles are sufficient to give an intense experience of the forehead with a quality of light. The second touch, at the end of the treatment, is merely a brief reminder of the first circles. The pentagram concludes with 1–3 circles in this area.

The ankles, at the other end, are markedly less sensitive. It will usually take 10 circles to help the mind to focus on this region.

The wrists are between forehead and foot also as regards sensitivity. Seven circles will usually be enough.

Do you use binding and relaxation dynamics when making the circles?
These dynamics are very much held back. The circles are flowing – without pressure, and sucking if possible. Suction quality arises as you inwardly let go, a quality that calls for special skill. Binding, or increasing intensity, and relaxation are qualities that come in mainly as the hand approaches and is taken away again. The flowing circles are like water poured into a basin that comes to rest after going round a few times. The relaxation is like the water evaporating in the warmth.

In which direction do the circles go?
On the forehead, they go anticlockwise, which is the direction in which the procedure then continues. On the extremities, the circles follow the way from the periphery to the heart, i.e. anticlockwise on the right foot and right hand, clockwise on the left foot and left hand.

What role does the free hand play during the Einreibung?
As the Einreibung is done with one hand, the question arises as to what the other hand is doing. It is not moving but attentive. It does not touch the patient, nor does it hold the covers or tube of ointment. It describes an arc which is open towards the patient.

6.3   Mood and inner attitude

Extreme concentration is needed to reduce the field of treatment to five very small areas. Too much pressure, movements that are too quick, sudden touch or letting go, 'angular' circles, confusing the sequence of areas to be treated, restless steps in walking around the bed, etc. all affect the subtle web of touches made.

Patients are not generally used to having their forehead and heart touched and it does intervene in a highly personal sphere. The utmost respect is therefore called for.

Concentration on the quality of touch and the progress of the treatment, and on active respect for the patient's boundaries only seems possible if the carer directs the whole of his attention to perceiving the treatment sites. Moving from one point to the next, the carer should come upright, walk in a measured step, and keep the whole pentagram in mind.

Being a mediator in bringing in etheric forces from the periphery when approaching and making contact, and then going out to the periphery when letting go and moving on to the next treatment site – this is the inner rhythm experienced by the carer.

6.4   Indications

As the pentagram has a special relationship to the human ether body (see Background, 6.1), and because of the character of the immediate experiences and effects of the pentagram Einreibung, we can establish three groups of indications (Table 3.1).

6.4.1   Questions concerning the indications

How often should a pentagram Einreibung be done?
As a rule the first two treatments are the most intensive. Many patients are then able to reac-

tivate the harmonizing principle merely by calling the Einreibung to mind again. A sequence of three consecutive Einreibungen would therefore appear to be sufficient in most cases. The treatment may be repeated after some days. One treatment a week will often be sufficient.

Which substances may be used?
Ointments and oils are generally suitable. Gold ointment (Aurum metallicum prep.) has proved effective in supporting the rhythmical to and fro between incarnation and excarnation and strengthening the I-middle, which are the two typical indications for the pentagram Einreibung. It is in the nature of this metal to combine maximum density with the most luminous lustre, earth and heaven, in harmony. This makes it an effective image and archetype for the integrative powers of the human middle (the I). The ointment contains gold in potentized form. A very good combination is of gold with lavender and rose (Aurum comp. ungt./ Weleda).

What are the contraindications?
Nothing is known so far about the treatment being unsuitable for particular patients. Caution is, however, indicated with schizoid psychotic patients. The marked introversion which may result may lead to inner experiences they are unable to control.

Table 3.1 Indications and examples of the pentagram Einreibung	
Indication	Examples
Conditions of being frozen in body and in dissolution in the psyche	anxieties, depression, rheumatic conditions
States of physical dissolution, with the psyche in a frozen state	certain stages in the dying process
Deterioration in the heart, the organ of the middle	cardiac failure, bradycardia, tachycardia
Supporting the original image of the human form for those with disabilities and deformation	physical development disorders in children, (congenital) disabilities, sclerosing conditions
Supporting the original physical and psychic integrity after severe stress or trauma and acute diseases	extreme exhaustion, in the puerperium, transitory syndromes following accidents or surgery, in convalescence

Can the treatment be given to unconscious patients?

It is not easy to establish if it has an effect with somnolent or comatose patients. The calming of respiration, pulse and blood pressure may, however, indicate that the Einreibung does also do something for them. Those with temporarily altered consciousness do often show significant improvement in mental clarity and orientation.

Is the treatment suitable for patients who are extremely restless?

Patients with motor unrest are not usually accessible for this treatment. If the restlessness does not die down as the Einreibung is done on the forehead, it is advisable to treat the feet with strong strokes on the soles.

Patients suffering from inner unrest, on the other hand, experience the marked concentration as a help in controlling their anxieties. This is a major indication for the pentagram Einreibung.

Can children be treated?

The treatment appears to be indicated especially for children with disorders affecting physical or mental development. It provides them with the very essence and archetype of physical and mental development.

Sources

Hauschka M. *Rhythmical Massage as Indicated by Ita Wegman.* London 1979.

Buehler W. *Das Pentagram und der Goldene Schnitt als Schoepfungsprinzip.* Stuttgart 1996.

7   *Monika Fingado*   Rhythmical Einreibungen of organs according to Wegman/Hauschka

Organ Einreibungen according to Wegman/ Hauschka (called 'Organ Einreibungen' below) are a special area in the field of Rhythmical Einreibungen. Here we enter into the world of internal organs and organic functions that govern all vital processes in the body and colour the life of the psyche. This is also the sphere for the actions of metals and planets which have an inner connection with these organ systems. Ointments containing metal preparations are therefore almost always used for organ Einreibungen. The cosmic dynamics that create our organs can thus shine into the organism through the gateway of the skin.

Simple forms are used for Organ Einreibungen. 'You might, of course, make warm circular movements everywhere, as these serve to bring things together inwardly,' and 'this can be enhanced by making the movement one that breathes' [Hauschka], e.g. with a lemniscate or by increasing and decreasing contact and inner binding and relaxation to give the movement the right rhythmical quality for the given organ. Form and rhythm address each organ with this 'gentle' form of massage, offering it the archetype of healthy function. This leads to a 'gentle awakening of the organ's function' [loc. cit.], a hint which continues to sound during the rest period which follows and which can initiate a healing process.

An Organ Einreibung takes about two minutes, after which you often sense that the organ has 'had enough'. If treatment continues for too long, the effect may be the opposite, the organ having been given more than it can cope with and unable to respond in a healthy way.

The methodology given so far for Rhythmical Einreibungen also applies to Organ Einreibungen. The latter are highly effective and deep-acting and need to be used in a very specific way, being aware of your responsibility. It is particularly important that they are only done by an experienced carer with a light hand using close contact, and that knowledge of the forces active in the organs and of the actions of metals gives rise to an inner image that stays with the carer during the treatment.

In this chapter, consideration of the organs and their functions and of their relationship to metallic and planetary processes can only cover the aspects relevant to understanding the Einreibungen. For further details, see the literature listed at the end. A brief description will be given of the Organ Einreibungen as they are done at the Ita Wegman Clinic in Arlesheim, Switzerland. The indications are many, and will be limited to some typical uses to serve as examples.

7.1   Liver Einreibung

The liver is our largest and heaviest digestive gland. Countless hexagonal hepatic lobules make up its soft, spongy tissue. Five different fluid streams provide the internal structure. The proportion of water is only slightly below that of blood. The liver can store a large volume of blood; it triggers the sensation of thirst [Steiner 1999], thus regulating the volume and composition of circulating blood. It is the chief organ in the water organism.

Water is the vehicle for life, the precondition for constructive etheric vital processes. The liver is our central metabolic organ and involved in almost every anabolic process, our vital organ in the vegetative sense. It plays a crucial role during embryonic development and in the first years of life when its size relative to body volume is much larger. The liver's detoxifying function is also constructive. Having enormous powers of regeneration, the organ is capable of creating new tissue from residual tissue remaining after surgical removal of parts of it, doing so within a few weeks.

Bile production is an integral part of liver function that goes in the opposite direction. Bile, one of the most aggressive body fluids, separates and degrades substances. The pigment which gives it its colour derives from the degradation of blood and thus contains the iron impulse of destroyed red blood cells. Bile enables us to digest the fats taken in with our food. The heat generated in the process provides a basis for physical activity.

Treatment of the hepatic and biliary system consists in evenly flowing circles over the right lobe of the liver, enveloping this area in warmth and giving impulses. It concludes with a brief, close and gentle down stroke. A possible image of this treatment would be the rings which an impulse creates on the surface of water.

Superficially, the Rhythmical Einreibungen of the liver does not differ from that of the gallbladder. The quality will be different, however, if treatment is given in a dreamingly unconscious, watery liver mood or else a rousing, fiery gall mood.

An Organ Einreibungen with tin ointment given in the evening will stimulate the constructive functions of the liver and may be used, for instance, to treat congestion or chronic hardening. Tin (Stannum), which relates to the planet Jupiter, is a soft, ductile metal with crystalline infrastructure. It remains in the fluid state between melting and evaporation for an unusually long time and creates order and form when processes are too fluid or if they have hardened.

Treating the liver with iron ointment in the morning, on the other hand, will address more the active biliary functions. Iron (Ferrum) is the metal of martial Mars, god of war. It gives human beings the energy to act, whilst lack of iron causes feebleness and exhaustion. Thus we can give an impulse that will wake up, strengthen the will, and so stimulate the power to make decisions and be active, for instance in case of depression, tiredness and lack of drive after hepatitis or when people are inwardly resigned in the face of life's challenges.

7.2   Kidney Einreibung

Human kidneys are about the size of a palm and 'typically kidney-shaped'. Their highly dif-ferentiated internal structure presents a very different image compared to the liver. The two kidneys form a pair but are not entirely symmetrical in position and size. They are located in the abdomen but behind the peritoneum. One side is unbroken and rounded, the other open, with a concavity and the afferent and efferent vessels and ureters. Kidneys have a cortex and medulla, elongated tubules and vascular glomeruli, with marked differences in pressure and an enormous throughput of fluids. The 150 litres of primary urine produced daily are reduced by active resorption, resulting in a daily output of between 1 and 2 litres.

The kidneys thus have numerous properties that are polar opposites, and this suggests air in motion, able to play between the extremes of stillness and gale force. The astral element of the soul also lives in the airy sphere and we can see other relationships to it in the kidney.

These organs are highly sensitive to pain. Their function is not 'dreamily unconscious' like that of the liver; urinary excretion increases with stress or when we are too wide awake. The soul connects with the body via the renal system.

The kidneys eliminate the nitrogenous products of protein catabolism (urea and uric acid). Nitrogen, the main constituent of the ambient air (79 %), is a constituent of protein and therefore an important building stone in the ensouled animal and human body. The kidneys may be called the organ of the airy principle. They control the lungs' respiratory functions via the acid-base balance and are therefore connected with air hunger.

To treat the kidney, make calm, warming circles over each kidney region. Let your hands always go across to the other side after some circles. This creates a connecting lemniscate. To conclude, do a warmth circle encompassing both kidneys and a delicate, soft downstroke towards the sacrum. In accordance with the airy nature of the kidney, do this Einreibung with a bit of a swing, almost dancing, and let it be light and rhythmical.

We generally use ointments containing copper (Cuprum), the Venus metal. This is a soft metal of reddish, warm colour and a full, warm sound. It warms through and nourishes. A treatment given in the morning can counter and reduce excessively destructive, catabolic day-time activities for people who are extremely nervy and therefore rather weak. In the evening the treatment can help the soul to come free of the body.

7.3   Heart Einreibung

The heart is the centre of our circulatory system. It is a 'meeting place', where currents of blood at different temperatures and with different oxygen and nutrient levels come together. Blood from the lungs brings the impressions gained through contact with the outside world to it and these are different from those which the blood brings from 'the small world of our own inner organism' [Steiner 1983].

In the constantly repeated, steady alternation between contraction and relaxation, blood from the peripheral circulation collects in the heart before every beat. It comes to rest for just a moment before it spreads out again into the extensive network of capillaries. The heart thus mediates between inside and outside, receiving and letting flow, coming to itself and going out into the world with the courage of the heart.

The heart is not only our centre in physical, bodily terms, but also holds a central position, we feel, in the psyche, where we connect it with warmth and inwardness, courage and strength.

Treating the heart, we make a large circle, very calm, in steady flow, over the left chest, going beyond the upper body. It is important to convey a wide expanse when letting go, taking with it all that inwardly oppresses and constrains. Nor should any pressure be exerted over the mid-chest. An inner free space can arise.

Gold (Aurum), the metal we use with heart treatments, belongs to the Sun, the 'external heart' in our planetary system. It has a noble lustre, is immune to outside influences and acts to restore equilibrium and fill the human being with light.

Treating the heart has a calming and strengthening effect with nervous palpitations and nervous heart trouble and when one lacks courage to face up to difficult situations in life.

7.4   Spleen Einreibung

The spleen is an elastic blood sponge. Contractile arteries allow it to regulate its blood volume, and the organ swells up some hours after food has been taken. Because of the pulsating variation in size it has been called the 'elastic heart of the vascular system' [Rohen 2001]. It functions in its own rhythm.

The spleen has a high proportion of lymphatic tissue and therefore plays an important role in immune defences and immuno-tolerance, being able to recognize and deal with foreign substances that may prove harmful to the organism (e.g. incompatible substances or bacteria). The spleen is one of the few organs that can apparently be removed without serious consequences. The operation is merely followed by reduced immunotolerance and a greater risk of infection.

Rudolf Steiner spoke of the spleen as an organ where our organism borders on the outside world, its true function being to balance out irregular food intake and the regular rhythm of the blood, 'changing the rhythm', as it were, of the foreign substance so that it may be integrated in our own rhythm. In a way this is therefore another immunological function, though less firmly bound to the physical, bodily organ. In this sense the spleen is a 'very spiritual organ' [Steiner 1999].

Treatment of the spleen consists in a large, rhythmically highly differentiated lemniscate. One loop is done with full, warm contact of the hand over the region of the spleen. Inwardly we relate wholly to the organ as we do it. With the other, small loop, which may be 'almost contracted into a turning point that is breathing' [Hauschka], we go far out inwardly, as if we wanted to take new impulses from the Saturn sphere and give them to the organ.

Lead (Plumbum), the metal most widely used when treating the spleen, belongs to Saturn, the planet which marks the boundary from our solar system to the rest of the cosmos. It is a dark, heavy metal which shields from radiation, sound, heat and explosions.

The treatment can help patients who are too open and unprotected as well as those who are too closed up on themselves to find the right kind of boundaries. It may thus be used for patients with neurodermatitis, numerous food intolerances and allergies.

7.5   Liver and spleen Einreibung

In conclusion I'd like to refer to a special treatment suggested by Rudolf Steiner. It consists in treating the liver with iron ointment and the spleen with copper ointment in the mornings. 'Massage of the liver sets old karma from the past in motion again, and massage of the spleen allows karma to find the right configuration for the future' [Deventer 1992]. The iron impulse strengthens the will, helping to break open a past that has hardened too much, inwardly work through it and accept it; copper gives warmth, making it possible to receive new impulses for the future in loving warmth and making them part of oneself.

'For most patients, the primary cause lies here, and Ita Wegman would therefore prescribe this external application very frequently' [loc. cit.].

Sources
Deventer MP van. Die antroposophisch medizinische Bewegung in den verschiedenen Etappen ihrer Entwicklung. *Natura*. Arlesheim 1992.

Hauschka M. *Rhythmical Massage as Indicated by Ita Wegman*. London 1979.

Holtzapfel W. *Im Kraftfeld der Organe*. Dornach: Verlag am Goetheanum 2000.

Husemann W. *The Anthroposophical Approach to Medicine*. Vol. 1. Tr. P. Luborsky. Spring Valley: Anthroposophic Press 1982.

Rohen J. *Funktionelle Anatomie*. Schettauer Verlag 2001.

Steiner R. *Introducing Anthroposophical Medicine*. Tr. J. E. Creeger. Hudson: Anthroposophic Press 1999.

Steiner R. *An Occult Physiology*. London & New York: H. Collison & Anthroposophic Press 1932. 3rd ed. London: Rudolf Steiner Press 1983.

Treichler M. *Sprechstunde Psychotherapie*. Stuttgart: Urachhaus 1993.

Chapter 4
Practical exercises
Hermann Glaser

It is only through the morning gate of the beautiful that you will enter into the land of insight.

... for the route to the head through the heart must be opened up. The more urgent need in our time is thus to develop powers of sentience and feeling....

Friedrich von Schiller

Nur durch das Morgentor des Schönen
Dringst du in der Erkenntnis Land.

... weil der Weg zu dem Koft durch das Herz muss geöffnet werden. Ausbildung des Empfindungsvermögens ist also das dringendere Bedürfnis der Zeit....

Friedrich von Schiller

The practical exercises discussed in this chapter may be done individually or by groups in training courses. They provide a basis for developing the quality needed for Rhythmical Einreibungen. The aim is to let central elements come alive in experience. Having developed the necessary awareness, it will then be easier to integrate them in the procedures.

The exercises are designed to awaken the will to learn in a living, artistic and playful way, and to get you in the way of asking questions. 'Aha' experiences that fire enthusiasm are the carrot, as it were, that will make you want to take the subject further. Beginners have often been known to have an original, intuitive feeling that arouses their curiosity and motivates them to become actively involved.

I have tried to select simple exercises that will set you on the way, ultimately helping you to be creative and develop your own. Variations are possible with most of the exercises, making repetition interesting and lively. Practice leads to progress. With every repetition, new windows and doors open up, and the panorama before you grows wider and wider.

Many of the exercises have been collected and formulated by my colleagues in the Rhythmical Einreibungen trainers' group at the Filder Clinic.

Rhythm is the repetition of something similar.
Johann Wolfgang von Goethe

Rhythmus ist Wiederholung des Ähnlichen.
Johann Wolfgang von Goethe

1   Methodology

All method is rhythm. Having the rhythm of the world, you also have the world. Every person has his own individual rhythm.
A sense of rhythm is genius.

Novalis

Alle Methode ist Rhythmus: hat man den Rhythmus der Welt weg, so hat man auch die Welt weg. Jeder Mensch hat seinen individuellen Rhythmus.
Rhythmischer Sinn ist Genie.

Novalis

1.1   Preparation

The stiffness must go, with rule being no more than the hidden baseline when we do things in a living way.

Johann Wolfgang von Goethe

Das Steife muss verschwinden und die Regel nur die geheime Grundlinie des lebendigen Handelns werden.

Johann Wolfgang von Goethe

First of all, a suitable setting must be created.

The room must have a pleasant, friendly atmosphere. Blend out possible disruption coming from outside and have the necessary materials to hand.

Before you start, be clear about the rules of the game. Will people be allowed to talk or should silence reign? How is the group organized in the given space – in pairs or groups of people? How much time will you have?

It is important to give an outline of the exercise, speaking of the aim, the meaning and purpose without pre-empting the result. The inner eye must be given an orientation if the exercise is to bear fruit.

Writing some key terms on the board may help people to remember.

If you sense incomprehension, ask if anything is not clear. Uncertainty and failure to understand are inhibitive.

You can help people to have the necessary self confidence and to be motivated by using humour to encourage, offering support if there are difficulties, acknowledging the existence of inhibitions, and taking people and what they say seriously.

1.2   Execution

Endeavour to make beauty the mediator of truth, and with that truth to give beauty a permanent basis and greater dignity.

Friedrich Schiller

Man wird streben, die Schönheit zur Vermittlerin der Wahrheit zu machen, und durch die Wahrheit der Schönheit ein dauerndes Fundament und eine höhere Würde zu geben.

Friedrich Schiller

You need to develop a feeling for the right length of an exercise. People lose interest if it takes too long, and they cannot have the experiences that will allow them to formulate concepts if it is too short.

There should be no pressure to succeed. The exercises need to be done in a completely relaxed way. This will create a climate where new ideas, skills, and also a degree of community spirit can develop.

It is important to pay attention to things said, done and experienced.

Feelings will often arise that point to important learning aspects. You cannot dispute them but must take them seriously and let them be expressed.

Warm interest, marvelling at the phenomena, will help us relate to the subject. Enthusiasm arising at this point will prove infectious! At the same time it may also be necessary to maintain something of a cool distance to have the right relationship to the content.

At this point, questions have to be asked: What caught my attention? What was not so good for me?

1.3   Evaluation

Beauty is ... the rhythmical movement, harmony, or I don't know what to call it, between two people, person to person, between mind and feeling, between the rest and motion which the universe, world history, life — if we consider it quietly ... and strongly — make known to our heart and mind. Within a limited compass it is something to be seen in every work of art. All and sundry have part in this spirit, the soul of the universe, when connecting their life with the whole. Each must to the best of his ability let receptivity for its revelations come alive and grow.

Adam Mueller

Die Schönheit ist ... jene rhythmische Bewegung, Harmonie oder, wie soll ich sie nennen, zwischen zweien, zwischen Mensch und Mensch, zwischen Geist und Gefühl, zwischen Ruhe und Bewegung, die das Universum, die Weltgeschichte, das Leben, wenn wir es mit Stille und Kraft ... betrachten, unserm Gemüt mitteilt; und welche in beschränktem Umkreise jedes Kunstwerk darstellt. Dieses Geistes, der das Universum beseelt, ist alles und jedes teilhaftig, was sich mit seinem Leben an das Ganze anschließt, und die Empfänglichkeit für seine Offenbarungen muss jeder in sich beleben und erhöhen, wie er vermag.

Adam Mueller

Start with a short pause, to help concentration.

Was the atmosphere cheerful, tense, busy, reserved or boisterous?

Only go into details relating to individual groups once people have formulated their results, or if they have problems in putting them into words.

People often feel a bit uncomfortable if each is asked to say something in turn. The method is relatively effective but may cause people to cook something up on the spot, just to let the next person have their turn.

It is better if you manage to talk about it in a relaxed way, asking that everyone should take part. Good humour can be very encouraging here. Questions which demand more than a Yes or No for an answer are most likely to take things forward. At the least, every Yes or No should be followed by going further into it or giving an example.

Questions like
Did I have 'Aha' or 'Oh dear' moments?
What did I perceive, see, hear, ...?
What went on inside me at the time?
What was a problem?
What did become clear?
       will elicit answers beginning with
I found that ...
I was surprised to ...
I liked it that ...
The most important thing, I felt, was ...
I'd like to know if ...
I ask myself why ...

It is often helpful to express experiences in images. As you compare, weigh, deepen, work through the different aspects in lively discussion, seeking to come to the essence — an abundance arises that may initially seem confusing, but ultimately yields nourishment rich in essence.

Summing up at intervals can assist in keeping to the point, giving others the opportunity to add something.

Write the results up on the board, especially if they will be the basis for course material to follow. You can then always refer back to them.

Unclear statements will actually help things forward on occasion, but you need to pay attention to dependent clauses or problems with the formulating or development of concepts and try to go through it together.

It is also perfectly alright to show that for the moment you are unable to understand something someone has said. Letting a good question stand, asking everyone to look for an answer as the work goes on, strengthens the learning atmosphere.

Gradually you will be making some of those many things your own. New feelings and thoughts begin to arise. Or perhaps also questions or wishes. With each of them another seed is germinating, one that may prove fruitful for you. Others continue to lie dormant. At this point it is a good idea to make some notes, summing up how far you have got. What have I learned so far that is important? What do I want to follow-up further?

How the results apply in the sphere of Rhythmical Einreibungen should be as easily understandable as possible. A language rich in images is most likely to prove helpful.

As the training course progresses, you may refer again and again to the experiences people gained and this will have a degree of resonance, so that the qualities we seek to develop are made our own at a deeper level.

Make sure the evaluation is not more long-winded than your introduction. You want the most important points to be remembered rather than get lost in a welter of information.

2 List of the exercises given

Exercises for individuals
- Exercises to train the hands, our 'instrument' for Einreibungen
  experience of lightness or buoyancy (basic exercises)
  being alive yet inwardly relaxed
  intensity of contact (basic exercises)
- Perceptiveness in the encounter
- Room for play where tension is concerned (basic exercises)
- Study of relaxed hands in art
- exercises to get your hands warm.

Exercises done in a group
- Exercises for a sense of form
  - walking forms in space (basic exercises)
  - blackboard drawings with straight lines and curves.

Exercises for quality of touch
- 'Tutti-frutti' – different ways of touching and their effect (basic exercises)
- Shaking hands
- Touch to make the encounter
- Raising a hand with a specific idea and intention
- Unambiguity of touch

Exercises in technique
- Balancing – for a flexible posture
- Wrestling – for a flexible stance and relaxed attitude (basic exercises)

- Rolling off someone's back – for flexible mobility
- Throwing balls – for preparing to move
- Experiencing touch – to make controlled contact
- Exercise for ongoing awareness (basic exercises).

Exercises in sensory perception
- Exploring objects by touch blindfolded
- Hand impressions (basic exercises)
- Who am I?
- Sensing the presence before touching.

Rhythm exercises
- Passing balls around in 'short-long' rhythm
- Beat and rhythm (basic exercises)
- Rhythm and 'Sensitive Chaos'
- Pendulum swing
- Breathing exercise: tensing and relaxing, moments of reversal (basic exercises)
- 'Letting go inwardly' – with the fist as example
- Rod exercise in a circle
- Moments of reversal in space
- Looking at pictures and objects with reference to the substance question and the subject of rhythm.

3   Exercises for individuals

These exercises make it possible to gain new insights and make them your own in the classic sense — by constant repetition. Good habits develop, grow into abilities and skills at our disposal, and finally mature. Constant practice takes things to the point where they come naturally.

It is often also possible to develop such exercises step by step.

Most are quite short and can be practised again at odd moments.

> Love life even in its most inconspicuous aspects and you will bear witness to it all the way, even where your most inconspicuous movements are concerned.
>
> Christian Morgenstern

> Habt das Leben bis in seine unscheinbarsten Äußerungen hinab lieb, und ihr werdet bis in eure unscheinbarsten Bewegungen hinab unbewußt von ihm zeugen.
>
> Christian Morgenstern

3.1   Exercises to train the hands

> Palm
> inside of the hand.
> A sole that goes on no more than feeling.
> Facing upwards and receiving heavenly streets in the mirror — walking themselves.
> Knowing how to walk on water when it goes to draw it,
> walking on the wells,
> changing all pathways.
> Appearing in other hands,
> making her ilk into landscape —
> wandering and arriving in them,
> filling them with arrival.
>
> Rainer Maria Rilke

> Handinneres
> Inneres der Hand.
> Sohle, die nicht mehr geht als auf Gefühl.
> Die sich nach oben hält und im Spiegel himmlische Straßen empfängt, die selber wandelnden.

> Die gelernt hat, auf Wasser zu gehen, wenn sie schöpft,
> die auf den Brunnen geht,
> aller Wege Verwandlerin.
> Die auftritt in anderen Händen,
> die ihresgleichen zur Landschaft macht:
> wandert und ankommt in ihnen,
> sie anfüllt mit Ankunft.
>
> Rainer Maria Rilke

3.2   Experience of lightness or buoyancy

Aim
Do this exercise for some time and you'll be surprised how sensitive you've become to the power which water has to uphold, its buoyancy.

Description
Attentively touch a water surface and slowly enter into the water through its 'skin'. The hand experiences the 'suction' as it connects with the surface tension – similar to the tone of our skin. Let the mid-hand experience itself as the centre in this play of forces.

Opportunities for practice arise all the time – when you wash in the morning, wash the dishes, bathe the children, and why not also when there's such a tempting big puddle in the meadow?

3.3   Being alive yet inwardly relaxed

> The senses are the bridge from the incomprehensible to the comprehensible.
>
> August Macke

> Die Sinne sind die Brücke vom Faßbaren zum Unfaßbaren.
>
> August Macke

Aim
To feel your hands come alive again. Recalling this 'state of bliss' will prove immediately

helpful when you want to 'remind' your cold, clumsy hand of the need to relax when doing an Einreibung.

Description

Young children like to stroke velvety soft kittens, let fine sand run through their fingers, put warm mud into the 'little bowl' of their hand. Tension in the hands will relax spontaneously. A smile appears. This means that the pleasure and enjoyment is flowing through the whole organism. Such fine and subtle stimuli, kind to the hand, develop it into a keenly perceptive organ.

Discover it for yourself again.

3.4   Intensity of contact

Aim

This exercise develops familiarity with intensity of contact in a Rhythmical Einreibung.

Description

Put a terry towel on a smooth surface (table, chair, grand piano or similar). Try and pass your hand across it very lightly and yet richly.

The material will throw folds or travel across the surface – too strongly!

The towel does not move but tickles your hand – too lightly!

Imagine your hand to be a leaf which the wind is moving across a calm pond. Observe carefully how the water bears the leaf. Connect with it (do not float above it).

3.5   Perceptiveness in the encounter

Every movement of the hand can cause separation or mean union.

Marta Heimeran

Jede Bewegung der Hand kann trennen oder einen.

Marta Heimeran

Aim

Here you discover that touching another person with sensitive awareness can be something that develops trust, reflecting and addressing the essential nature of that other individual.

Description

When did you last consciously shake hands with someone?

Make it your intention to do so. Pay attention to the tension that meets you.

Is the other person's hand listless or does he hold yours in a tight grip?

Watch how your hand responds. Does it take hold of the other person, or does it shrink back?

Ideally sympathy develops as you shake hands, more like a 'dance' of the two hands. The tension in the hand will move between being light and then again firm. There will be time to note if the other hand is warmer or cooler than your own, damp, rough, narrow or rather large and heavy.

3.6   Room for play where tension is concerned

Aim

The following exercise will give better control of alternating tension and relaxation in the hand. It will then be easier to find the right moment for relaxation during an Einreibung.

Description

Slowly and in full awareness close your hand to make a fist. Then open up again, paying careful attention to the sensations in the hand.

Repeat a number of times and then try to open up a fist energetically, maintaining the tension. The hand should open up again even so. It will, but it is almost torment and results in a twisted claw hand.

Deliberately turn off this 'high tension' now and ... lo and behold: the hand is able to open up like a flower in the sun. Enjoy the relief! Repeat this process as well, inwardly growing aware of the brief moment when you resolutely turn from tension to relaxation.

3.7   Study of relaxed hands in art

Beauty comes when you sense rhythm.

Christian Morgenstern

Schönheit ist empfundener Rhythmus.

Christian Morgenstern

Aim

The aesthetics of relaxed hands can be found in the arts. This awakens a feeling for the subtle play of muscles which permits all and every intention to come to expression through the human hand.

Description

Look at hands making harmonious gestures in sculptures, drawings or paintings. See if you can describe what makes a hand look beautiful. Try and put your own hand in the same position.

3.8   Exercises to get your hands warm

Aim

All exercises designed to train hand skills will in the long run also help to make constitutionally cold hands warmer.

Sensory perception plays a major role in this and with it, the opening and relaxation of the hands, i.e. their responsiveness.

There will, however, be situations where inner tension and nervousness suddenly make the hands go frozen again. Every trainer has known this to happen when giving a demonstration before a large group of strangers. Many carers know it when asked to do an Einreibung in the busy turmoil of ward life. Below are some tips which everyone may try for themselves until they find their own way of getting hands warm quickly.

Description

Try to put your two hands together in such a way that the hollow between them is a sphere.

Let the mid-hands be relaxed as they feel their way to the inside of the sphere, go back again a little, pulsating, and so on.

Let one, two or three smallish wooden balls roll around in your hands – forward, back, sideways – then also in circles to the left or right. The increased sensitivity and mobility of the hands will cause them to warm up.

An earlier exercise was playing with water. You will draw warmth to your hands more quickly and lastingly with warm water than with the dry heat provided by a hot-water bottle. Washing the dishes can also be a good way of preparing to do an Einreibung. Making a ginger or yarrow compress for one patient before giving an Einreibung to another will also let your own hands have the benefit of these warming substances. If all else fails, it will help to go to the washbasin and let a gentle stream of warm water flow on to the inner aspect of the wrists and from there over the hands. The developing quality of your touch will be altogether enriched if you grow sensitive to the movements of water, bearer of life and responsive to rhythm, meditatively taking them in and letting them come alive in you.

You will find that warmth begins to flow after just a few Einreibung movements that have been given a definite rhythm. So if you don't want to shock the patient with your 'icicles', you might make a few movements over the shirt or the cloth or towel covering him. Or spoil a colleague on the ward with a few strokes down her stressed back before you hurry on to the patient – two minutes will be all that is required.

Woollen wristlets, whilst not an exercise, can however be a help during the period of preparation. They aid relaxation in the wrist, an area where the flow of warmth often tends to be blocked.

4   Exercises done in a group

The overriding aim with these exercises is to let group members experience new qualities in their actions, learning by making their own discoveries. They can then also discover the laws and apply them in their work with Einreibungen.

Group exercises also create a common 'feeling' – team spirit. This will also help individuals to cope better with the challenges met in the course. The feeling of being part of a group sustains them.

4.1   Exercises for a sense of form

4.1.1   Walking forms in space

If you develop a feeling for form, for things you can see, you will gradually enter into an inner mood where ideas come as the occasion demands.
Rudolf Steiner

Wenn man für Formen, für Anschaubares Sinn entwickelt, dann lebt man sich allmählich in eine Seelenstimmung hinein, bei der einem etwas einfällt, wenn Veranlassung dazu da ist.
Rudolf Steiner

Aim
Many people find it easier to do a form on the small scale, using their hands, once they have walked that form a few times.

Description
Walk in a circle (on your own or the whole group), with one person in the middle experiencing the process from the centre.

You might let the circle become a lemniscate, for example, and then add a whole sequence of walking exercises for certain aspects of this form:

a)   Everyone walks in a circle (following one another)
    1   round the circle (fairly fast)

2   crossing in zip-fastener mode (∞) (easing up on the pace)
3   with the right arm outstretched
The arm – and your attention with it – will point to the periphery on one side and inward on the other (conveys a feeling for alternation between expansion and concentration). In one loop you gather together what is received from outside or let go to the outside in the other.

b)   Each walks a vertical lemniscate on his own (facing forward)
If you go clockwise through the loop in front, you will be going anticlockwise in the one at the back.
Again polarities are conveyed.
Walking the form dynamically you feel the urge to go faster along the straight parts. In the curves, however, you tend to walk more slowly, with circumspect attentiveness.
Walking a horizontal figure of eight facing forwards, you follow axial symmetry in moving through the two loops. Here it is possible to get a feeling for an element of weighing things up, balancing them out.

c)   Two people going in opposite directions walk a horizontal figure of eight. They start from opposite extremes and move at a steady pace at first and then, on the inside, faster and closer. You will experience inner oppression as you become aware of the crossing point as the most dynamic element. It is important to take courage and give clear form to the point of intersection. This is also a good way of giving people the experience of circles with phase shift, with two people representing the left and right hand respectively, and a third the spine, walking backwards bit by bit (down the back, as it were). All are walking backwards. This calls for great awareness of what is happening around one.

All other Einreibungen can also be made visible in space, moving on the large scale. If the group is large enough, it is even possible to create a large-scale image of a whole-body Einreibung.

It is advisable to walk always facing forward, i.e. facing the same wall (the hands will later also be required to move in a resting position).

In every instance, dynamic aspects may be added as a further element, alternating between speeding up and slowing down once the form is clear in everyone's mind.

4.1.2   Blackboard drawings with straight lines and curves

... equally far from monotony and confusion dwells the form that wins the day.

Friedrich Schiller

... gleich weit von Einförmigkeit und Verwirrung ruht die siegende Form.

Friedrich Schiller

Aim
To develop a feeling for the quality of these form elements, which will then be rediscovered in the Einreibungen.

Description
Ask the group to create a picture on the board, using different colours.

For the first attempt, they should use only perfectly straight lines, Let each draw a line of any length in a place where they feel something is still needed to achieve a harmonious whole. This continues until all are agreed that the picture is finished.

If it is possible to cover the drawing up and leave it until a drawing using curved lines has been produced at the next session, a comparison of the two can prove very instructive.

5   Exercises for quality of touch

5.1   'Tutti-frutti' – different ways of touching and their effect (basic exercises)

Aim

This exercise takes you into the world of touch as the most elementary approach to another human being.

You learn how touch of different quality always has a specific effect.

Description

Let people try out every possible way of touching the back of a partner – rubbing, for instance, patting, pinching, towelling, kneading, circular movements, quiet or rapid strokes, striking with the edge of the hand, with and without change of direction.

Ask them to observe the effect of angular and round, large area and point wise, rapid and peaceful, firm and light movements, as well as those going from below upwards, from the outside to the inside, and vice versa.

List the results on the blackboard under the headings 'pleasant' and 'unpleasant', always defining the statements, e.g.

- flowing, circular movements (relaxing)
- short, difficult contacts/tickling (incalculable, restless > goose bumps)
- light touches with the whole hand (more intensive)
- too much pressure (heavy, oppressive)

You learn to use touch in a controlled way if you know what a particular touch feels like. You may then ask yourself: What does this patient need? What do I want to achieve with him, and how can I do this?

It is important to realize that a sick person will react with much greater sensitivity than someone taking the course.

People also need to be aware that some qualities listed as rather unpleasant can on occasion be felt to be absolutely positive and used to good effect, among them the pressure on acupressure points to relieve a headache.

5.2   Shaking hands

Aim

The central aspect of this gesture is perception of one self or I by another. Eye contact is part of this, as is facial expression and perhaps a few words. You are always revealing something of yourself and perceiving something of the other individual.

Yet it is not only the handshake which tells something about us, but also our hands in themselves and what they do. We need to be aware of this when working with sick people.

Description

Shaking hands is one way in which one person greets another. You briefly want to meet the other in a more personal way than by merely saying Hello.

Get the group to try out every possible way of shaking hands. A 'normal' handshake, a very firm one, a loose one ('kiss of a cloud'); or you only let the other person have your fingers; or you won't let go ('vice'); pulling the other hand towards you or pushing it away; taking the other hand in both your hands.

5.3   Touch to facilitate a meeting

Aim

Certain regions of the body are highly sensitive and private. We are naturally hesitant to touch them.

Conscious experience gained in this exercise should help carers to use the necessary caution and distance in approaching the other person when doing a chest or abdominal Einreibung.

Description

Ask members of the group to draw someone's attention to themselves by touching them in some way or other, making contact with them and creating a meeting.

Let them sit in a circle. The exercise is to be done by each in turn, so that everyone is observing how one of them touches his neighbour. End with a general discussion.

5.4 Raising a hand with a specific idea and intention

Aim

Members of the group perceive that there are different ways of consciously guiding the effect of a touch. Describing these in relation to the qualities of the four elements will help to apply these in practice.

Description

Each individual in turn is to take up his neighbour's hand which is resting on the thigh, and with a short treatment express the idea that the hand appears to be cold, painful or lifeless. A fourth possibility would be to investigate where a cut or something like it may be found.

There follows a round where first the observers and then the person treated say what they thought it was, with the person who did the treatment confirming or correcting. The group will then try and characterize the different qualities of touch. Images from the realm of the four elements can be helpful with this, for instance the enveloping 'broodiness' of a hand that warms, the airy 'blowing away' of pain, or the gently flowing way of elevating to lightness in case of oedema or a stroke.

5.5 Unambiguity of touch

Aim

It will immediately be obvious how and where touch has reality or remains unreal.

Description

An exercise in pairs. One lies on the floor. The other is asked to get him upright. Not a word to be said. The person lying on the floor is allowed to move only as much as is clearly signalled by touch.

Success demands enormous empathy and decisiveness on the part of the leader, and the most careful attention on the part of the one lying down, listening to the hands of the other.

6   Exercises in technique

6.1   Balancing – for a flexible posture

> Strength can be made up for by balance, and everyone should maintain balance, for this is really the state where he has freedom.
>
>   Novalis

> Stärke läßt sich durch Gleichgewicht ersetzen, und im Gleichgewicht sollte jeder Mensch bleiben, denn dies ist eigentlich der Zustand seiner Freiheit.
>
>   Novalis

Aim

Centre of gravity, shifting weight and balance are brought to experience.

Description

Rods are needed for this (wooden, if possible). Everyone is asked to balance the rod on different parts of the body:

*   Across a finger, then on the head
*   standing vertically on a finger (sometimes the right hand, sometimes the left, try different fingers), on the dorsum of the foot ...

6.2   Wrestling – for a flexible stance and relaxed attitude (basic exercises)

> Alternating binding and letting go helps freedom to develop.
>
>   Wilhelm Hoerner

> Wechsel von Bindung und Lösung fördert die Freiheit.
>
>   Wilhelm Hoerner

Aim

To develop awareness of stance and posture during an Einreibung. The more flexible and free the stance, the freer and more relaxed the movement. Just leaning against the bed with one leg, or supporting yourself on the bed by one hand will limit your movement.

Description

Working in pairs, people face each other, holding hands. By mutual agreement, one tries to upset the other's balance (taking turns), varying the stance:

1   with legs fixed, i.e. knees straight and feet firmly planted on the ground, going through different degrees of difficulty, for example:
    – feet in line (toes to heel, as if walking a tightrope)
    – feet close together (legs together)
    – one leg ahead of the other, as if walking. The exercise might also be done with the back straight and stiff. This will limit mobility further, the feeling of distance between the wrestlers increasing.
2   Using the legs in a flexible way and being fully mobile, all possible moves and change of step are now permitted.

Flexibility needs much space and freedom of movement and a calm middle sphere from which the connection to the area below is maintained and therefore the burden of gravity controlled. With one foot forward, you have a broad base area, with the weight well balanced between the leg carrying the weight and the other.

A variant of the exercise can make you aware of other aspects:

Two partners stand face to face, each with feet together, the distance between them such that they can reach the shoulder of the other with their fingertips.

The task is to upset the balance of the other by suddenly letting your hands shoot forward. It is important to have a well-aimed, straight forward impulse, and to have elasticity in the shoulder for defence.

You should be able to maintain your stance like a young bamboo shoot or a field of wheat.

Rigid trees will break or be uprooted! A free shoulder girdle is the centre for secure movement.

Durch gymnastische Übungen bilden sich zwar athletische Körper aus, aber nur durch das freie und gleichförmige Spiel der Glieder die Schönheit.

Friedrich Schiller

6.3   Rolling off someone's back – for flexible mobility

Aim
The aim is to develop conscious awareness of one's own back. We tend to forget about it because we are always looking ahead.

You will not only be more awake in your back, but also altogether more upright after every exercise.

It will also become easier to integrate the hollow of the back in the Einreibung gesture of being there for the patient.

Description
Two partners stand back to back and let their backs roll off each other. First from above downwards, then from below upwards to come upright again. Attention is mainly focussed on the backbone.

A 'hole' is created by the hollow of the back. Contact is apt to be lost at this level, but can be consciously established at this point by tilting the pelvis.

The exercise can be taken further by trying to go into a crouch, back to back, and then return to a standing position whilst still together.

Good collaboration is essential, otherwise the whole will soon be out of balance.

A further development of the exercise would be for a third person to put his hand at some point between the partners' backs. The two should then try to meet particularly at this point.

A similar exercise can be done on your own by lying on your back on the floor and endeavouring to connect the whole hollow of the back with the floor.

6.4   Throwing balls – for preparing to move

Gymnastic exercises will lead to the development of athletic bodies, but beauty only comes with the free and even play of the limbs.

Friedrich Schiller

Aim
Being able to walk upright, human beings can freely move their arms. They do not need them to support the body but can use them in many different and differentiated ways. With the greatest possible mobility in the shoulder girdle as well we are thus able to create rhythm out of lightness, buoyancy, when doing Einreibungen.

In everyday life we are not, as a rule, aware of this freedom of movement. The exercise is designed to bring these resources to mind and encourage carers to use the whole arm for Einreibungen.

Description
Each person has an elastic ball, the kind used for juggling or tennis (not wooden or copper, etc.).

Let them toss the ball to and fro between their hands or with a partner, but with the forearms held close to the hip, so that at first only finger and hand joints are mobile. The process is gradually made easier by freeing the arms from the immobility – first to the elbows (which means that now only the upper arms are firmly 'attached' to the flanks), and finally also to the shoulder joints.

Involvement of the shoulder girdle (shoulder joint, shoulder blade and clavicle) even in relatively small arm movement (turning the hand from prone to supine) can be brought to awareness with the help of a partner. His hand lying loosely on my shoulder blade will clearly perceive the subtle changes that occur, at the same time also making me aware of the region's involvement. The immediate consequence is that I can guide my arm in a more relaxed way.

6.5   Experiencing touch – to make controlled contact

Aim
Showing how light one's touch must be, and how low the tension, and that the touch can nevertheless be close or intense.

Description

Set up a training sequence

a) for contact
    – towel on a smooth surface (e.g. a table)
b) for a relaxed hand
    – piece of soft fur
    – bowl of warm water
    – fine sand
    – ball/balloon with soap or talc
    – unspun wool
c) for ongoing awareness
    – copper cylinder/bottle

First possibility

Let your hand move in a rich, full way on the towel without producing folds in it. This gives you the quality of snugness for stroking or effleurage over an area. If contact is so close that the towel begins to move around, you have gone beyond the level of intensity required, which is when the height of the crescendo has been reached in an Einreibung.

Second possibility

Let the hand move across the fur. Tension will go spontaneously. Contact is warm and snug.

Third possibility

Let the hand touch the surface of water and separate from it again. Forces of suction and lightness are experienced, being in 'conversation' with the tissue. Going deeper, you experience the buoyancy as the 'pressure' of water. At this point conversation may arise about how it feels when we immerse ourselves completely in water.

Fourth possibility

The hand moves gently and lightly on the surface of sand or you let the sand run through completely relaxed fingers.

Fifth possibility

Rub a ball or balloon all over with soap or talcum – initially following its form in a completely relaxed way. Later it will also be possible to use the exercise to practice ongoing consciousness or intensifying deep into tissue and the letting-go process which follows.

Sixth possibility

Try to tease unspun wool apart. This will only succeed if you do not tear at it but proceed gently and carefully in a relaxed way.

Seventh possibility

The exercise for ongoing awareness must have been done before this (6.6).

You can let your hand roll over a copper cylinder or a bottle, first without relaxing the hand (like a board), then with the hand relaxed.

Further thoughts on the above may be found in Section 3.1 (Exercises to train the hands).

6.6   Exercise for ongoing awareness

Aim

The exercise is a great help in getting a clear idea of how this activity of the mind goes hand in hand with Rhythmical Einreibungen.

Description

Everyone is asked to look for an easily accessible seam in the clothes they are wearing and see if they can sense the seam as the hand moves lightly and slowly across it, initially from finger pads to heel of hand and vice versa, and then perhaps also across the hand, with the parts of the hand which have passed over the seam relaxed and loose. You can test this by using the other hand to play with the fingers (are they stiff or mobile?) or moving the wrist a little bit (building up a bit of tension only in the place of contact with the seam). A good image for this is one of countless eyes in the hand which are open or closed – awake in the region of attentiveness, and otherwise asleep.

Repeat the whole, but now on an imaginary seam.

Let the hand remain in place, and conscious awareness move around its margins. Do you sense roundness?

The exercise can also be done on a balloon or a bottle, and in this case you can look through this at the palm of your hand, with the wide-awake eyes in it almost tangible.

7   Exercises in sensory perception

7.1   Exploring objects by touch blindfolded

I see with my feeling eye, feel with my seeing hand.
> Johann Wolfgang von Goethe

Ich sehe mit fühlendem Aug, fühle mit sehender Hand.
> Johann Wolfgang von Goethe

Aim

The exercise makes us realize that in everyday life we do not go into our sensory perceptions but bar our own way to independent insight by being too quick in coming to conclusions. (What did the patient look like? Did he really look like that? Or does he merely look like that to me because he also looked like this yesterday?)

A thoughtless traveller and a scholar living in abstract notions are both unable to gain many and varied experiences.
> Rudolf Steiner

Der gedankenlose Reisende und der in abstrakten Begriffssystemen lebende Gelehrte sind gleich unfähig, sich eine reiche Erfahrung zu erwerben.
> Rudolf Steiner

Description

Each is given an object which he does not see and must explore by touch. The object should be one that is not too easily recognizable.

The aim is not to discover as quickly as possible what I have in my hand but rather to observe how I arrive at that discovery.

Do I start with details? The general impression? How does the idea gradually evolve? How much can I learn about the object if I let myself be wholly guided by the senses?

What is perceived more easily with which part of the hand? (Something heavy tends to lie in the palm; finely chiselled forms are explored with the finger pads.)

Another way is to start the exercise with the concept. Someone describes an object, the others form an idea, finally all objects are exhibited and considered.

7.2   Impressions given by hands

Aim

The aim is to base an opinion not only on visual perception but use also the potential of the other senses.

Eliminating the sense of sight means that we lose certainty, feel disorientated and hesitant. Trust is needed, and listening through touch assumes an important role.

Description

People move about the room with their eyes closed. Each finds a partner, or the group leader divides the group into pairs. None should speak, if at all possible.

Each then examines the partner's hands, taking time to do so. Tasks are set for this at intervals:

Compare the upper side and underside of the hand, i.e. the quality of the dorsum (bony, hairy), the muscles of the inside hand (hills and vales), or note the state of warmth, moisture, proportions (e.g. width of palm, length of fingers), the general configuration of the hand (form and size), the mobility of its parts.

What is the handshake like?

In conclusion, each forms an idea of the person belonging to the hand.

The members of the group are then asked to look at the hand with open eyes, and so the secret is revealed.

For a two-day course, the exercise could be extended as follows. Ask individual blindfolded members of the group to feel a number of hands and see if they recognize the hand from the day before.

A variant is to let a small group of about four people stand in a circle and consider, feel and compare the characteristics of the different hands, continuing with this until everyone feels they will be able to tell them apart. Then blindfold one member of the group and ask him to decide which hand belongs to which person just by feeling it.

7.3   Who am I?

Aim

This exercise makes you aware that the hand which touches holds a differentiated expression of the human being in it. A human being is speaking in that hand.

Description

It is important for the room to be quiet.

Make up groups of four. The four should be familiar with one another.

One person in the group turns his back on the others, closes his eyes and is now touched by the others, alternating between effleurage and a circling movement.

He must see if he can tell which 'Einreibung' was done by whom. What tells us who it is?

7.4   Sensing the presence before touching

If you do not venture beyond reality you'll never gain the truth.

Friedrich Schiller

...wer sich über die Wirklichkeit nicht hinauswagt, der wird nie die Wahrheit erobern.

Friedrich Schiller

Aim

The aim is to realize that a person's 'sphere' begins long before you are in touch with their physical boundary. This is important for any contact by touch in nursing.

The hands learn to listen.

Description

Two partners always sit facing each other. Closing their eyes, they move their palms towards one another. They need to concentrate and see if they can tell the moment when they sense the presence of the other and how this happens (warmth, a tingling, 'wall of air' or 'field of dust'?) Is there a gradual transition or a definite boundary?

Which part of the hand is most sensitive to perceptions of this kind?

The eyes may be opened as soon as the presence of the other is perceived, to check how far away he still is.

Close attention is needed. Without it you will continue to move until you make skin contact, not noticing anything before that.

8   Rhythm exercises

8.1   Passing round balls in 'short-long' rhythm

Aim

To practise moving between giving and receiving.

To take pleasure in rhythm, you must find your healthy middle, not being too much in yourself yet also not losing yourself in the other.

Description

Everyone stands in a circle, each with a small ball in the hand (right or left hand for all). The group agrees on a rhythm, e.g. short-long. With 'short', the ball goes from a player's one hand to the other; with 'long', the ball is passed on to the next person. Depending on the rhythm, the direction may change when the ball is passed on (e.g. with short-short-long), or the balls continue in the same direction all the time.

All start together. The more practised people are, the more can the process be speeded up.

8.2   Beat and rhythm

Rhythms are life kept on the move in mind and spirit.

Igor Stravinsky

Rhythmen sind geistig bewegtes Leben.

Igor Stravinsky

Aim

Mainly to experience the qualities of beat, rhythm and chaos in play.

Description

Everyone stands in a circle. Initially all clap together as regularly and monotonously as possible. Then people clap in turn, to begin with once each. A direction has been agreed on. The volume of the sound should also be as even as possible.

Beat should result — a sequence of 'metronome-like' claps done as exactly as possible.

It is good to be a bit finickety over this, for the group will then on the one hand be able to learn how difficult it is to maintain the beat, and on the other to experience how an inner need arises to overcome the beat and be allowed to make things come alive.

Enforced tiredness and mild aggressiveness give way to pleasure and laughter when people are then permitted to

- reduce or perhaps also increase sound volume, taking some care (no break in the flow)
- pass the clap in a different direction by turning left or right
- or indeed throw it to someone across the circle, or
- produce 1, 2 or 3 claps on a beat.

Take care to catch the right moment for stopping the exercise before it slides into chaos. Though even then people will realize that a little chaos is more enlivening than being tied to a beat for a long time.

In conclusion the group clap together, first quietly in the beat, next increasing speed and volume until it becomes wild applause and then trying to find their way back to a quiet, regular ending.

8.3   Rhythm and 'Sensitive Chaos'

Pulsating in all and everything, losing your self to nothingness.

Christian Morgenstern

In allem pulsieren, an Nichts sich verlieren.

Christian Morgenstern

Aim

Primarily to generate rhythm deliberately.

The exercise may be used when you want to wake the group up and make them aware of their extremities.

Description

The group stand in a circle.

Give them a rhythm to clap that is not too complicated (e.g. long-short-short-long-long). It can help to give them a phrase in the rhythm: Klatsch in die Haende (now clap your hands, do).

The rhythm is to arise in that each does a particular number of claps and then the next person takes over.

The degree of difficulty can be increased in a number of ways:

- clapping only with the hands (in one direction), each doing one clap in turn.
- only stamping your feet (in one direction; starting with the right foot – i.e. going clockwise – appears to be easier for all right-handed people), each doing two beats.
- Each does three beats – right foot, hands, left foot (or in the opposite direction).

One problem is the difficulty in maintaining the rhythm at all. Too much concentration results in tension, breaking the flow as people come in too soon. Lack of attention leads to stops and starts, the whole slowing down. In either case, the next person will also be losing it. It can be a help if one person provides orientation by clapping the rhythm centrally throughout, or if the rhythm is also spoken.

8.4   Pendulum swing

Give as you receive, and learn to receive in your giving.

J. C. Lavater

Gib, indem du empfängst, und lerne im Geben empfangen.

J. C. Lavater

Aim

An exercise for courses designed to teach manoeuvres and Einreibungen for special medical conditions. It will help people to develop a feeling for states of sudden loss of stability (e.g. from shock) or spasticity and constriction (e.g. with asthma).

Description

Two partners let their hands come together (both or only the left or right hand) and try to find a rhythm as they swing to and fro. Suddenly and surprisingly one of them will upset the regular swing (as agreed beforehand). The other is asked to observe his reaction to this break in the flow of movement. The 'trouble-maker' can either give way completely, or get frozen or even hold fast to the other.

A shared pendulum swing should be regained after a short interval. The partners change roles after a while.

In the theoretical part which follows, consideration may be given to disease as loss of harmony, for instance when inflammatory metabolic processes or sclerotic tendencies from the neurosensory sphere overcome the middle, the rhythmical system.

In the first case, movements would lack definition, being wishy-washy; with the second one would get a mechanical to and fro, a kind of beat without pauses.

8.5   Breathing exercise: tensing and relaxing, turning moments

Aim

We find that a normal breath as it moves to and fro is far removed from the possible extremes of tension.

As with Einreibungen, problems arise when the processes of increasing intensity and relaxation are not kept cleanly apart. You will then either oppress the patient or make him 'breathless'.

Description

Ask the group to breathe in and out a number of times, doing so in full awareness.

We barely perceive the brief turning moments, though they are essential for rhythmical alternation. Initially those between inhalation and exhalation which call for an 'inward resolution' to let go – though at an unconscious level. Yet this alone will enable us to breathe out again. Then the moment which follows exhalation – one of absolute rest and relaxation before a new breath is taken.

The exercises allow us to experience what happens if these turning moments do not come. Ask the group to take a deep breath and then maintain the tensed posture as they try to breathe out again. This will only prove possible with the aid of the accessory breathing muscles that squeeze the air out. If you forget to pause after an exhalation, your breathing becomes hectic and panting, losing all rhythmical alternation.

Next ask the group not to exhale after taking breath, but continue to inhale for as long as possible. Then breathe out normally.

As a final step, ask them to inhale first, and then exhale to a maximum degree.

8.6 'Letting go inwardly' – with the fist as example

Tension is all, and release. And the highest
wisdom for life is always to release your tension
rightly.
                                    Christian Morgenstern

Spannung ist alles und Entladung. Und höchste
Lebensweisheit, seine Spannung immer richtig zu
entladen.
                                    Christian Morgenstern

Aim
It is important for the rhythmical quality of Einreibung-movement that the tiny moment of inwardly letting go is taken up consciously. The necessary 'remelting' process will then succeed in the inner turning moments of an Einreibung. Isometric release of the tension which has developed must go hand in hand with a change in quality.

Description
Let everyone concentrate on their hand, making a fist and then opening it up again. Is it possible to describe what went on inwardly? You can discuss the phases of tension and relaxation, referring to the same processes in breathing and other rhythmical processes.

How is the transition from tension to relaxation achieved? A familiar image is that of a monkey reaching through narrow bars to get a nut and being unable to draw its fist back, being unwilling to let go of the nut.

In the same way we cannot release a fist unless there is the inner resolution to let go – however unconscious it may be. The muscles go into spasm.

Let everyone try and open the fist whilst maintaining the same tension. It will not be possible to do better than a claw-hand.

Compare this to the relief experienced when the hand is decisively put in a relaxed position.

The tension can only go if something else happens. Just as the power of flexion changes to become a liberating force of suction when you open your fist, so does the tension at the high point of every Einreibung-movement of increasing intensity change to become warmth and lightness.

8.7 Rod exercise in a circle

Aim
Many of the elements of rhythmical activity come to experience, above all, relaxation in time without taking something along or dropping it – giving over at the right moment.

Description
The groups stands in a circle, each placing his or her rod vertically to make a circle in the middle. It is important to have individuals at a good distance from each other.

The task is to leave the rods standing as the members of the group move on. Someone says: 'Right', or 'Left'. Group members are only allowed to steady the rod with a flat hand, which they take away in an upward direction so that the rod does not get knocked over. They move in the indicated direction to the next rod, hoping it is still standing, so that they can take it over, the hand still flat.

8.8　Turning movements in space

The measure gives itself to the motion – the
response to forward being back,
and if this should create a stir, let calm then its
companion be.

Christian Morgenstern

Es teilt das Maß sich der Bewegung: dem Vor
erwidert ein Zurück,
und stürzt dich jenes in Erregung, gesellt ihr dies
der Ruhe Glück.

Christian Morgenstern

Aim

To experience that the quality of a turning
process is better for Rhythmical Einreibungen if
we manage to keep starting point and endpoint
in mind at the same time.

Description

Members of the group stand in two facing rows
with the whole width of the room between
them, each having a partner opposite.

Start by all walking forward in a leisurely way
until they are almost touching their opposites.
They then go back slowly to their starting point.
Let them pay attention to the processes of
approaching and then separating again. The
two lines should as far as possible stay in line,
as this will enhance the impressions to be
gained.

As you go on, let the lines move faster and
faster. The turning moment grows more and
more dominant: How do we avoid collision?
How can the movement still be flowing nevertheless?

To help them, each may imagine that a long
(rubber) band in the back connects them to
their starting point.

An interesting, more powerful variation is to
do the exercise with people walking towards
one another backwards. Additional aspects
concerning 'in front – behind' can be gained.
The region at the back of the neck then
becomes the organ of perception.

Let the group also try to do the same with
eyes closed, stopping when they feel that their
partner is getting close. It is remarkable how
sensitive one becomes as time goes on.

8.9　Looking at pictures and objects

Aim

To look at pictures and objects as a group can
help to convey quality concepts which are
otherwise difficult to present.

Description

'What spirit comes to expression in gold?' You
may follow this with the suggestion that before
they meet again everyone looks for a picture or
object that expresses the quality of gold. It may
be a picture of the mask worn by a Pharaoh, a
mosaic with gold background, an icon,
Rembrandt's *Man with the Golden Helmet*, or
perhaps just a simple wedding band. The group
will uncover many aspects, whereas a tutor on
his own would have difficulties presenting the
subject so comprehensively and clearly.

Or: 'What does copper have to do with the
kidney?' The attempt may be made to find an
answer by looking at Botticelli's *Birth of Venus*.
Someone might also tell the legend. In this way
members of the group will develop a feeling for
the relationships and grow curious about them.

For the subject of rhythm, group members
may bring along things that reflect an aspect of
rhythm for them.

9   In conclusion

Let me stress once again in conclusion that the exercises should be fun, but must also be taken seriously if they are to serve their purpose.

> It has been said many times that heroism may well be easier than slow, patient and unremarked self education, just as a deed may be easier than an action, a feeling easier than an inward response.
>
> Christian Morgenstern

> Wie mancher hat es schon ausgesprochen, daß Heldentum ebenso leichter sein kann, als langsame, geduldige, unauffällige Selbsterziehung, wie eine Tat leichter sein kann als eine Handlung, ein Gefühl leichter als ein Empfinden.
>
> Christian Morgenstern

Errata — notes

Since the publication of this book in German the need for adjustments to some of the diagrams and illustrations has emerged. The most important of these have been noted in the relevant places.

Fig. 9   The top circle on the right should be at the same height as the left circle.

Fig. 11   The blue hand should come more from the outside — thus following the curve of the arrows.

Fig. 12   The patient's hand should be covered and lie on the abdomen.

Fig. 15   The guideline (green) veers too much to the ventral side. It should follow the line of the muscle.

Fig. 18   The circle should be large enough to include the solar plexus.

Fig. 21   The last blue line should follow the guideline (green) off.

Fig. 26   The red dot should be lower, where the two balls of the foot are thickest.

Useful addresses

AMA (Anthroposophical Medical Association)
c/o Rudolf Steiner House
35 Park Road
London
NW1 6XT

Medezin Sektion
Goetheanum
Dornach
CH-4143
Switzerland
www.goetheanum-medezin.ch
sekretariat@medsektion-goetheanum.ch

The authors

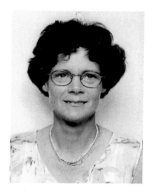

Monika Fingado, born 1956, trained as a nurse at Karlsruhe Municipal Hospitals, Germany; further training as nurse tutor at an institute for further and additional training in Unterlengenhardt, Germany; worked in a curative education home and various hospitals. From 1988 at the Ita Wegman Clinic, Arlesheim, Switzerland, nurse and tutor for in-house further training. Courses and publications on external applications, Rhythmical Einreibungen (Wegman/Hauschka) and other themes in anthroposophical nursing.

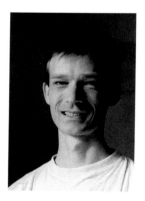

Hermann Glaser, born 1966, Abitur, non-military service (geriatric care) and training as a nurse; working at the Filder Clinic near Stuttgart, Germany, from 1990.

Took part in a practice-integrated study project for three years (caring relationships, external applications, form given to doctor's rounds, models for duty rosters, etc.), then became leader of an internal medical nursing team.

Apart from working as a nurse, he has been involved in further training work both in-house and at the clinic's school of nursing.

Practical tutor in Rhythmical Einreibungen (Wegman/Hauschka), giving public specialist courses and talks on external applications, Rhythmical Einreibungen and the anthroposophical nursing treatment of chronic ulcers.

Several publications on these subjects.

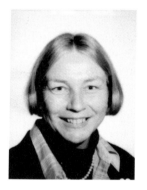

Edelgard Grosse-Brauckmann, RN, born 1944, trained as a nurse with the German Red Cross at Muenster/W. University Hospitals; nursing tutor, masseuse and medicinal baths expert, manual lymph drainage (MLD/KPE), practical tutor in Rhythmical Einreibungen (Wegman/Hauschka).

1969–1981, Herdecke Community Hospital (nursing on the wards, tutor and nursing management).

1982–1986, geriatric nursing (home and institutional care).

1986–1995, lecturer at institute for further and additional training in geriatric and general nursing (Verband anthroposophisch orientierter Pflegeberufe e.V., Bad Liebenzell, Germany).

From 1996, developing concept for training in Rhythmical Einreibung (Wegman/Hauschka) and giving courses on Rhythmical Einreibungen and the training of trainers in

Austria, England, Georgia, Germany, Russia, Sweden, Slovenia and the USA.

Working as a nurse for a few months/year at different hospitals.

Rolf Heine, born 1960, trained as a nurse at the independent school of nursing attached to the Filder Clinic near Stuttgart, Germany. Worked as a nurse in internal medicine, surgery and geriatrics. Tutor in nurses' training.

Involved in conception and implementation of a practice-integrated nursing research project for external applications and nursing relationship.

Since 1993 working in further training for nurses, and nursing advice with the emphasis on anthroposophical nursing. Also working in quality management and developing a curriculum for integrated anthroposophical nurses' training. Publications in books and journals on the following themes: inner development for nurses, body care, preventive measures, nursing relationship, nursing gestures, working with the dying, spiritual ethics.

From 2000, coordinator of International Anthroposophical Nursing Forum in the Medical Section, School of Spiritual Science, at the Goetheanum, Dornach, Switzerland.

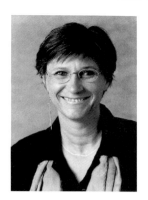

Monika Layer, born 1957, diploma in nursing, Berlin 1978; nursing tutor, Bad Liebenzell, Germany, 1987; consultant for organizations and supervisor, Grueningen, Germany, 1999.

Many years' practical nursing experience in intensive care, medical wards, rehabilitation and oncology in Germany and Switzerland, partly in leading positions; 1987–1992, tutor and head of independent school of nursing at the Filder Clinic, Germany; from 1993, tutor, lecturer, counsellor and coach in training, further and additional training for nurses in Switzerland; experience in processes of change with the restructuring/re-orientation of nursing diploma training courses; collaboration on a number of projects, incl. a practice-integrated nursing research project at the Filder Clinic, monitoring projects for the development of the training course for trainers in Rhythmical Einreibungen (Wegman/Hauschka); public lectures and courses in external applications and Rhythmical Einreibungen (Wegman/Hauschka); author of a number of publications.

Index